Rous Sarcoma: Current Research. I.

Papers by
Peter Duesberg, Warren E. Levinson, Howard
M. Temin, John P. Bader, Anthony Faras,
Axel-Claude Garapin, Lois Fanshier, Saiji
Yoshii, Alice Golde, Paul P. Hung, Christina
M. Scheele, R. L. Stolfi, Clifford J. Bellone,
Frieda K. Roth, G. F. Rabotti, Richard G.
Olsen et al.

MSS Information Corporation
655 Madison Avenue, New York, N. Y. 10021

Library of Congress Cataloging in Publication Data
Main entry under title:

Rous sarcoma: current research.

   1. Rous sarcoma. I. Duesberg, Peter.
[DNLM: 1. Sarcoma, Experimental--Collected works.
2. Rous sarcoma--Collected works. QZ 345 R863]
RC262.R68   616.9'94   72-10910
ISBN 0-8422-7063-9

TABLE OF CONTENTS

CREDITS AND ACKNOWLEDGMENTS

Bader, John P., "Synthesis of the RNA of RNA-Containing Tumor Viruses," *Virology*, 1970, 40:494-504.

Bader, John P.; and Nancy R. Brown, "Induction of Mutations in an RNA Tumour Virus by an Analogue of a DNA Precursor," *Nature*, 1971, 234:11-12.

Bellone, Clifford J.; and Morris Pollard, "A Transient Cytotoxic Host Response to the Rous Sarcoma Virus-Induced Transplantation Antigen (34851)." *Proceedings of the Society for Experimental Biology and Medicine*, 1970, 134:640-643.

Duesberg, Peter; Klaus V. D. Helm; and Eli Canaani, "Comparative Properties of RNA and DNA Templates for the DNA Polymerase of Rous Sarcoma Virus," *Proceedings of the National Academy of Science*, 1971, 68:2505-1509.

Duesberg, Peter; Klaus V. D. Helm; and Eli Canaani, "Properties of a Soluble DNA Polymerase Isolated from Rous Sarcoma Virus," *Proceedings of the National Academy of Sciences*, 1971, 68:747-751.

Duesberg, Peter; G. Steven Martin; and Peter K. Vogt, "Glycoprotein Components of Avian and Murine RNA Tumor Viruses," *Virology*, 1970, 41:631-646.

Fanshier, Lois; Axel-Claude Garapin; Jerome McDonnelo; Anthony Faras; Warren Levinson; and J. Michael Bishop, "Deoxyribonucleic Acid Polymerase Associated with Avian Tumor Viruses: Secondary Structure of the Deoxyribonucleic Acid Product," *Journal of Virology*, 1971, 7:77-86.

Faras, Anthony; Lois Fanshier; Axel-Claude Garapin; Warren Levinson; and J. Michael Biship, "Deoxyribonucleic Acid Polymerase of Rous Sarcoma Virus: Studies on the Mechanism of Double-Stranded Deoxyribonucleic Acid Synthesis," *Journal of Virology*, 1971, 7:539-548.

Golde, Alice, "Radio-Induced Mutants of the Schmidt-Ruppin Strain of Rous Sarcoma Virus," *Virology*, 1970, 40:1022-1029.

Hung, Paul P.; Harriet L. Robinson; and William S. Robinson, "Isolation and Characterization of Proteins from Rous Sarcoma Virus," *Virology*, 1971, 43:251-256.

Levinson, Warren E.; J. Michael Bishop; Nancy Quintrell; Jean Jackson; and Lois Fanshier, "Synthesis of RNA in Normal and Rous Sarcoma Virus-Infected Cells: Effect of Bromodeoxyuridine," *Virology*, 1970, 42:221-224.

Levinson, Warren E.; Harold E. Varmus; Axel-Claude Garapin; and J. Michael Bishop, "DNA of Rous Sarcoma Virus: Its Nature and Significance," *Science*, 1971, 175:76-79.

Olsen, Richard G.; James R. McCammon; Joseph Weber; and David S. Yohn, "Cutaneous Skin Test for Delayed Hypersensitivity in Hamsters to Viral Induced Tumor antigens," *Canadian Journal of Microbiology*, 1971, 17:1145-1147.

Rabotti, G. F.; and F. Blackham, "Immunological Determinants of Avian Sarcoma Viruses: Presence of Group-Specific Antibodies in Fowl Sera Demonstrated by Complement-Fixation Inhibition Test," *Journal of the National Cancer Institute*, 1970, 44:985-991.

Roth, Frieda K.: Paul Meyers; and Robert M. Dougherty, "The Presence of Avian Leukosis Virus Group-Specific Antibodies in Chicken Sera," *Virology*, 1971, 45:265-274.

Scheele, Christina M.; and Hidesaburo Hanafusa, "Proteins of Helper-Dependent RSV," *Virology*, 1971, 45:401-410.

Stolfi, R. L.; Ruth A. Fugmann; J. J. Jensen; and M. M. Sigel, "A C1-Fixation Method for the Measurement of Chicken Anti-Viral Antibody," *Immunology*, 1971, 20:299-308.

Temin, Howard M.; and Satoshi Mizutani, "RNA-dependent DNA Polymerase in Virions of Rous Sarcoma Virus," *Nature*, 1970, 226:1211-1213.

Yoshii, Saiji; and Peter K. Vogt, "A Mutant of Rous Sarcoma Virus (Type O) Causing Fusiform Cell Transformation (35039)," *Proceedings of the Society for Experimental Biology and Medicine*, 1970, 135:297-301.

PREFACE

The first oncogenic virus to be discovered, RSV remains a major focus of interest for those concerned with the etiology of cancerous growth. At present, RSV represents the best experimentally accessible model of an oncogenic RNA virus whose effects can be observed both *in vivo* and *in vitro*.

The present two-volume collection includes papers published from 1970–1972 on host cell surface changes induced by RSV, on the enzymic machinery contained in the virion as well as on the viral nucleic acids. Current research on RSV mutants or genetic variants is also presented.

NUCLEIC ACIDS OF ROUS SARCOMA VIRUS

Comparative Properties of RNA and DNA Templates for the DNA Polymerase of Rous Sarcoma Virus

PETER DUESBERG, KLAUS V. D. HELM, AND ELI CANAANI

Indirect evidence suggests that RNA tumor-virus replication requires virus-specific DNA early in infection (1, 2). This virus-specific DNA is thought to be transcribed from viral RNA by the virus-associated DNA polymerase (3, 4). The ubiquity of this enzyme in all known RNA tumor-viruses (3–5), its ability to transcribe *in vitro* most or all viral RNA (6, 7), and the presence of at least one enzyme per virion (8) are compatible with its role of a RNA–DNA transcriptase essential for virus replication. Very different kinds of nucleic acids, however, were reported to be templates for virus-associated DNA polymerase, perhaps indicating that Rous Sarcoma Virus (RSV) DNA polymerase is not specific for virus replication. Unpurified DNA polymerase of RNA tumor-viruses was shown to accept exogenous natural DNA (9–11), synthetic DNA, DNA–RNA hybrids, or double-stranded RNA as templates (10, 12) besides the endogenous viral RNA (4, 3, 6). Synthetic homopolymer RNAs, however, were found to be poor templates (12, 10), except when present with a complementary oligodeoxynucleotide primer (13). A purified DNA polymerase of RSV that was free of endogenous template responded to both natural DNA and single-stranded RNA templates, and preferred among natural RNAs the 60–70S RNA of RSV (8).

Abbreviations: RSV, Rous sarcoma virus; TMV, tobacco mosaic virus.

The present report describes quantitative comparisons of the template activities of various nucleic acids in the presence or absence of oligodeoxynucleotides for the purified RSV DNA polymerase. Further, the question of whether RNA and DNA templates compete for the same RSV DNA polymerase was investigated.

MATERIALS AND METHODS

[^{3}H]dCTP, [^{3}H]dTTP, 14–20 Ci/mmol; [^{3}H]dATP, 6 Ci/mmol were purchased from New England Nuclear, [^{3}H]dGTP 3 Ci/mmol from Amersham, deoxynucleotide triphosphates from Sigma or CalBiochem, and oligodeoxyribonucleotides (of chain length 12–18) from Collaborative Research Inc., Waltham, Mass. Poly(dAT) was a gift of Dr. M. Chamberlin.

Viruses. Prague RSV of subgroup (14) C was used to prepare (8) 60–70S RNA and DNA polymerase, unless otherwise indicated. DNase treatment of RSV RNA (8) was in 5 mM MgCl$_2$–5 mM KCl–50 mM Tris (pH 7.4). Schmidt–Ruppin RSV of subgroup A, myeloblastosis-associated virus of subgroup B, and avian leukosis MC-29 virus of subgroup A were all originally obtained from Dr. P. K. Vogt (14) and grown as described (8).

Standard DNA Polymerase Assay. Purification of the soluble RSV DNA polymerase (8) was in a 20–40% (v/v) glycerol gradient. The enzyme was stored at $-20°C$ in the gradient solution after the addition of glycerol to a final concentration of 50%.

Standard assays were at 40°C for 2 hr in 100 μl of solution containing 50 mM KCl, 50 mM Tris (pH 8.0), 5 mM dithiothreitol, 6 mM MgCl$_2$, three unlabeled dNTPs at 0.1 mM, and one [^{3}H]dNTP at 1.25 μM (8). The assay contained 15 μl of enzyme solution. Given a 20-fold purification of the enzyme, based on the total soluble protein of the virus (8) and the assumption that 2 A_{260} (measured in 0.2% sodium dodecylsulfate) of purified virus corresponds to 1 mg of protein (8), the protein content of 15 μl of enzyme solution was 50–75 ng, which was operationally defined as one protein unit.

RESULTS

Dependence of DNA synthesis on enzyme and template concentration

Constant concentrations of 60–70S RSV RNA, heat-dissociated RSV RNA (15), influenza RNA, or tobacco mosaic virus RNA were incubated with different concentrations of RSV DNA polymerase. Maximal [^{3}H]DNA synthesis was obtained in all cases with 2 protein units of enzyme (Fig. 1), 5 times more DNA was synthesized at saturating

11

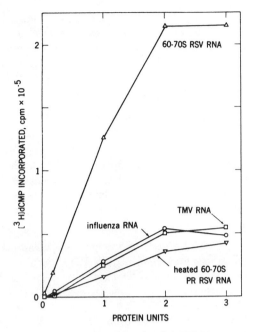

FIG. 1. Dependence of RNA-primed [³H]DNA synthesis by RSV DNA polymerase on enzyme concentration. 1 μg of the indicated RNA was incubated under standard assay conditions, but with different amounts of protein units (*Methods*) of purified enzyme.

concentrations of enzyme with 60–70S RSV RNA than when heat-dissociated RSV RNA or other RNAs were used as templates. This result is compatible with the hypothesis that a defined structure of the RNA template determines the rate of [³H]dCTP incorporation by RSV DNA polymerase.

Saturation quantities of a constant concentration (half-saturating for 1 μg of RNA, see Fig. 1) of RSV DNA polymerase with several nucleic acids are shown in Fig. 2. It appears that all nucleic acids reach, or at least approach, plateaus of maximal DNA synthesis at concentrations of 1–5 μg. Particularly with TMV RNA, but also with 28S ribosomal RNA and influenza RNA (Fig. 2B), the saturation curves suggest that there is inhibition of the enzyme by high concentrations of RNA templates. Heating of ribosomal RNA to 100°C, followed by sedimentation, did not affect its template activity, (not shown). Among the RNAs, 60–70S RSV RNA stimulates incorporation of [³H]dCTP 5- to 10-times better than all single-stranded RNAs tested, including heat-dissociated RSV RNA. The template activity of denatured salmon DNA (8) was about 1.3 times, and that of poly (dAT) about 3 times (see below), higher than that of 60–70S RSV RNA.

12

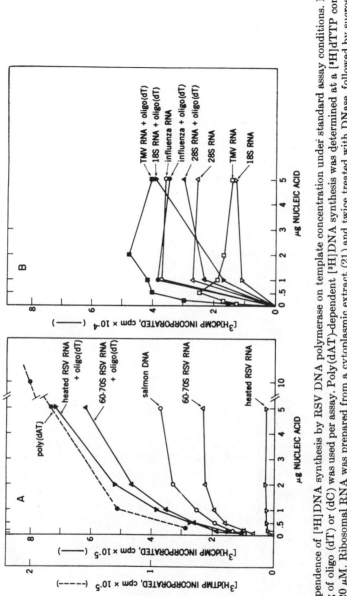

FIG. 2. Dependence of [³H]DNA synthesis by RSV DNA polymerase on template concentration under standard assay conditions. If indicated, 1 μg of oligo (dT) or (dC) was used per assay. Poly(dAT)-dependent [³H]DNA synthesis was determined at a [³H]dTTP concentration of 20 μM. Ribosomal RNA was prepared from a cytoplasmic extract (21) and twice treated with DNase, followed by sucrose gradient sedimentation.

13

Kinetics of DNA synthesis with several RNA templates

The kinetics of DNA synthesis with several RNA templates are shown in Fig. 3. All RNAs with high template activities, like 60–70S RSV RNA or RNAs in the presence of oligodeoxynucleotides (see below), exhibit relatively high rates of DNA synthesis early, and decreasing rates of DNA synthesis late, in an assay period of 2 hr. Heated RSV RNA stimulates DNA synthesis at a lower rate than does 60–70S RSV RNA, but the kinetics are similar to those obtained with 60–70S RSV RNA.

The kinetics of DNA synthesis with TMV RNA and 28S ribosomal RNA, however, show an initial lag period, but are otherwise similar to those obtained with the other RNAs. Despite these differences, the kinetics of DNA synthesis with various RNA templates are considered to be similar enough to justify a comparison of their template activities for RSV polymerase on the basis of the DNA yield that is obtained under standard assay conditions.

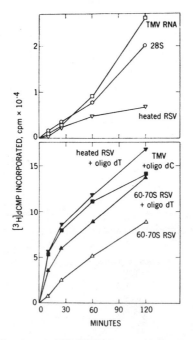

Fig. 3. Kinetics of [³H]dCTP incorporation by RSV DNA polymerase with 1 μg of the indicated RNA templates. 1 μg of oligodeoxynucleotide was added when indicated.

14

DNA polymerase of	RNA template	[³H]dTMP incorporated cpm
SR RSV-A*	SR RSV-A*	4804
	PR RSV-C†	3312
PR RSV-C†	PR RSV-C	62798
	SR RSV-A	48170
	MC29-A§	50852
	TMV	4826
MC29-A§	MC29-A	11402
	PR RSV-C	13862
	SR RSV-A	14374
	TMV	573
MAV-B‡	MAV-B‡	6322
	PR RSV-C	10271
	MC29-A	10782
	SR RSV-A	5005
	TMV	455

0.5 μg of template 60–70S tumor virus RNA or TMV RNA was assayed under standard conditions. Various amounts of enzymes were used, and are not equivalent for different viruses.

* Schmidt-Ruppin strain, subgroup A.

† Prague strain, subgroup C.

‡ Myeloblastosis-associated virus, subgroup B.

§ Avian leukosis virus, subgroup A.

Comparisons of the template activities of the RNAs of different avian tumor viruses

To determine whether the template activity of 60–70S RNA (Prague strain) for its homologous DNA polymerase was strain- or subgroup-specific (14), or whether all avian tumor virus RNAs have the same template activity for a given avian tumor virus DNA polymerase, the comparisons summarized in Table 1 were made. It can be seen that within the limits of accuracy of such assays, all 60–70S avian tumor virus RNAs have very similar template activities for a given enzyme.

Effects of oligodeoxynucleotides on template activities for RSV DNA polymerase

As shown in Figs. 2 and 3 and Table 2 the template activities of natural RNAs were increased by oligo(dT) or oligo(dC) 1- to several-fold. The template activity of heat-dissociated RSV RNA was increased 20- to 30-fold by oligo(dT) or by oligo(dC), and about 10-fold by oligo(dG). Oligo(dA) did not affect the template activity of heated RSV RNA. It appears that oligo(dT) or oligo(dC) restore the high template activity of RSV RNA that is lost after heat-dissociation to about the template activity of native 60–70S RSV RNA

TABLE 2. *Effects of oligodeoxynucleotides on the template activities of RSV RNA or KOH-denatured salmon DNA for RSV DNA polymerase under various conditions*

Standard assay* with indicated [³H]dNTP	Template (1 μg)	Oligo (dN) (1 μg)	[³H]dNMP incorporated, cpm (average ± range)§
	60–70S RSV RNA	. . .	103,850 ± 7000
	heated RSV RNA	. . .	7,200 ± 500
[³H]dCTP	same	(dT)	185,060 ± 12000
	same	(dA)	7,800 ± 800
	same	(dC)	257,081 ± 30000
	same	(dG)	72,508 ± 2050
	. . .	(dC)	434
[³H]dTTP	60–70S RSV RNA	(dT)	333,990 ± 16250
same	same	. . .	107,510
same	. . .	(dT)	1,030
same, −dATP	60–70S RSV RNA	(dT)	110,216 ± 4900
same, −dATP	same	. . .	500
[³H]dTTP†	poly(dAT)‡	. . .	108,405
same, −dATP	same	. . .	500
[³H]dCTP	60–70S RSV RNA	(dT)	42,056 ± 5000
same, −dATP	same	(dT)	306
same, −dTTP	same	(dT)	270
[³H]dGTP	same	(dT)	7,532
same, −dTTP	same	(dT)	219
[³H]dATP	same	(dT)	32,375 ± 450
same, −dTTP	same	(dT)	1,012
same, −dGTP	same	(dT)	822
[³H]dTTP	salmon DNA	. . .	76,226 ± 800
same	same	(dT)	79,480
same, −dATP	same	. . .	7,733

* The activities per unit of protein of different polymerase preparations varied about 2–3 fold in different experiments.
† [³H]dTPP was 2.6 μM, dGTP and dCTP were omitted.
‡ 0.3 μg. § of two determinations.

16

in the presence of oligo(dT) (Fig. 2). The template activity of TMV RNA was slightly stimulated by oligo(dT), but was stimulated about 10-fold by oligo(dC) (Fig. 3). Preliminary analyses indicate that the sizes of the DNAs produced in the presence or absence of oligodeoxynucleotides are similar.

About 1 μg of oligo(dT) per standard assay was necessary to maximize DNA synthesis directed by 1 μg of RNA template (experiments not shown). Oligo(dT) or oligo(dC) with-

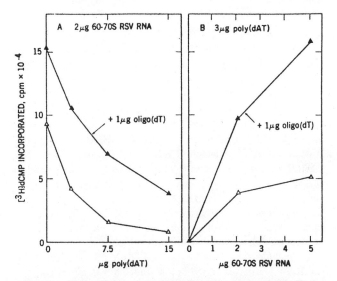

Fig. 4. Competition of 60–70S RSV RNA and poly(dAT) for RSV DNA polymerase. *A*. RSV RNA-dependent [³H]DNA synthesis was determined under standard assay conditions in the presence of 2 μg of 60–70S RNA, with or without oligo(dT), and different concentrations of poly(dAT), *B*. After incubation of RSV DNA polymerase for 30 min with 3 μg of poly(dAT) in a standard assay solution at 40°C, incubation was continued for 2 hr after the addition of various concentrations of 60–70S RNA, with and without 1 μg of oligo (dT).

out RNA (Table 2) or added after RNase treatment of a RNA template (not shown) did not function as a template for DNA synthesis. Oligo(dT) did not affect the template activity of KOH-denatured salmon DNA (8) (Table 2) or poly(dAT) (not shown).

Results of substrate deletion experiments are summarized in Table 2. RSV RNA-dependent DNA synthesis, measured by incorporation of [³H]dTTP in the presence of oligo(dT), was inhibited 70% if dATP was omitted. RSV RNA-dependent DNA synthesis in the absence of oligo(dT), as well as poly(dAT)-dependent DNA synthesis, were inhibited

17

99.5% if dATP was omitted, thus indicating that the [³H]-dTTP was not contaminated by dATP. If RSV RNA-dependent DNA synthesis in the presence of oligo(dT) was measured by incorporation of any of the other three [³H]dNTPs, however, there was 97% inhibition if an unlabeled dNTP was omitted. These results are compatible with the synthesis of a T-rich polydeoxynucleotide as well as virus-specific DNA (7) in the presence of 60–70S RSV RNA and oligo(dT), and imply that there may be an A-rich sequence of RSV RNA.

Amount of [³H]DNA synthesized in the presence of various templates

Under standard assay conditions, the amount of [³H]DNA formed (at a counting efficiency of 25% for ³H) by RSV DNA polymerase, relative to the 60–70S RSV RNA template, was 4–6%, and as much as 12% in the presence of oligo(dT) or oligo(dC) (Figs. 1 and 2, Table 2); it doubled if the molarity of [³H]dCTP was raised from 1.25 μM to 50 μM (not shown). With TMV RNA, ribosomal RNA, or influenza virus RNA, [³H]DNA synthesis was $\leq 1\%$ relative to the template added; more DNA was made in the presence of oligo(dT) or oligo(dC) (Fig. 2). DNA synthesis with a poly(dAT) template was about 50% or more at a [³H]dTTP concentration of 26 μM (Table 2). Since the above estimates were obtained at high or saturating concentrations of enzyme, we can conclude that the amount of DNA formed relative to the RNA templates added is low under our conditions.

Competition of RNA and DNA templates for the DNA polymerase

To test whether RNA and DNA templates compete for the same RSV DNA polymerase, the following experiments were done. [³H]DNA synthesis was measured in the presence of constant, saturating (Fig. 2) amounts of 60–70S RSV RNA, with and without oligo(dT), and with different concentrations of poly(dAT). Only RSV RNA-dependent DNA synthesis is measured by incorporation of [³H]dCTP, although poly(dAT) is an excellent template for RSV DNA polymerase (Fig. 2) (16). As shown in Fig. 4A, increasing concentrations of poly(dAT) reduced incorporation of [³H]dCTP into [³H]DNA. Further, if different concentrations of 60–70S RSV RNA were added to a standard assay solution during 30 minutes of poly(dAT)-dependent DNA synthesis, incorporation of [³H]dCTP into [³H]DNA increased (Fig. 4B). These results indicate that 60–70S RSV RNA, particularly in the presence of oligo(dT), can displace poly(dAT) from RSV DNA polymerase, and that both templates have similar affinities for the enzyme.

18

DISCUSSION

The finding that poly(dAT) inhibits RSV RNA-dependent DNA synthesis by RSV DNA polymerase is consistent with the hypothesis that RNA- and DNA-dependent DNA syntheses are performed by at least one common active site of the same enzyme or enzyme complex. This result is compatible with previous observation that RNA- and DNA-dependent polymerase activities of RSV coincide in sucrose gradients (8) and phosphocellulose columns (v. d. Helm, unpublished). It is possible, however, that RNA- and DNA-dependent DNA syntheses occur at different active sites, and that DNA acts as a template at one site and blocks RNA-dependent DNA synthesis at the other.

It seems likely that the increase of template activities of RNAs with oligo(dT) or oligo(dC) is due to their interaction with the RNA template. This can be deduced from the observations that oligo(dT) or oligo(dC) are, by themselves, without significant template activity and have different effects on the template activities of different RNAs. Further work will be necessary to decide whether oligo(dT) and oligo-(dC) interact with complementary regions of the RNA template, as suggested by analogy to the experiments of Baltimore and Smoler (13), or whether there is also some interaction with the enzyme.

As a tentative explanation for the results that at (probably) saturating concentrations of the enzyme (Fig. 1), or of RNA template (Fig. 2), 60–70S RSV RNA has a 5- to 10-fold higher template activity for RSV DNA polymerase than do heat-dissociated RSV RNA and the other RNAs tested, the following hypothesis may be suggested. Two different types of RNA structure determine the template activity of a given RNA: partially double-stranded regions, which probably exist in 60–70S RSV RNA (15) or hybrid regions, which might exist in the presence of oligodeoxynucleotides, are required for optimal binding to the enzyme and serve as optimal starting points; they thus account for the high rate of DNA synthesis. Certain regions in single-stranded RNAs, such as a self-complementary loop, may resemble partially double-stranded RNA and stimulate DNA synthesis at a lower rate. The low yields of DNA synthesis obtained even with high concentrations of single-stranded RNAs may be due to enzyme inhibition. At high concentrations of single-stranded RNA, the enzyme may not be permitted to transcribe a maximal region of the RNA template, because it may be displaced (e.g., Fig. 4) by binding sites of an RNA that is unable to initiate DNA synthesis. Partially double-stranded regions may also account for the high template activities of denatured salmon-DNA or poly(dAT).

19

It is conceivable that with partially double-stranded RNA, one strand serves as a template and the other as a primer, which may be incorporated in the DNA product. Preliminary experiments on characterization of DNA product obtained with 60–70S viral RNA as template after brief synthesis (unpublished) suggest that at least some DNA product is covalently linked to RNA after velocity or isopycnic sedimentation in 1.1 M CH_2O. These results are compatible with those of D. Baltimore and J. Hurwitz (personal communication).

An interpretation of the result that low amounts of DNA are formed by RSV DNA polymerase relative to the RNA templates tested cannot as yet be given. It may be due in part to an obligatory primer requirement.

The template requirements of RSV DNA polymerase suggest that the enzyme resembles bacterial DNA polymerase, which is known to prefer a partially double-stranded DNA template (17) and to transcribe single-stranded DNA optimally in the presence of an oligodeoxynucleotide primer (18). However, bacterial DNA polymerase, which has been shown to accept RNA templates (19, 13, and 22), and RSV DNA polymerase may differ with respect to template specificities for RNA.

The essential question as to whether RSV-associated DNA polymerase is involved in virus replication (4, 3) cannot be answered definitively on the basis of its known *in vitro* properties. Some properties that favor its role as a replicase are listed in the introduction. Other *in vitro* properties of the enzyme, including the relatively low synthesis of DNA with the RNA templates tested and the rather small sizes of the *in vitro* DNA products (20, 6, 10), do not support its putative role of a virus-specific RNA–DNA replicase, but these properties may be due to experimental artefacts of the *in vitro* systems.

NOTE ADDED IN PROOF

An adenylate-rich region has been found in RSV 70S RNA (M. Lai, unpublished data).

We thank Drs. W. M. Stanley and H. K. Schachman for encouragement, Drs. P. Berg, H. Rubin, G. S. Martin, M. Chamberlin, and T. Hurwitz for discussions, and Drs. Baltimore and Smoler for a preprint of their paper. Marie Stanley gave excellent assistance.

This investigation was supported by research grant CA 11426 from the National Cancer Institute and by Cancer Research Funds of the University of California.

1. Temin, H. K., *Proc. Nat. Acad. Sci. USA*, **52**, 323 (1964).
2. Duesberg, P. H., and P. K. Vogt, *Proc. Nat. Acad. Sci. USA*, **64**, 939 (1969).

3. Baltimore, D., *Nature*, **226**, 1209 (1970).
4. Temin, H. K., and S. Mizutani, *Nature*, **226**, 1211 (1970).
5. Schlom, J., D. H. Harter, A. Burny, and S. Spiegelman, *Proc. Nat. Acad. Sci. USA*, **68**, 182 (1971).
6. Duesberg, P. H., and E. Canaani, *Virology*, **42**, 783 (1970).
7. Duesberg, P. H., P. K. Vogt, and E. Canaani, ed. L. G. Silvestri, 2nd Lepetit Colloquium, on *The Biology of Oncogenic Viruses* (North-Holland 1971), p. 154.
8. Duesberg, P. H., K. v. d. Helm, and E. Canaani, *Proc. Nat. Acad. Sci. USA*, **68**, 747 (1971).
9. Spiegelman, S., A. Burny, M. R. Das, J. Keydar, J. Schlom, M. Travnicek, and K. Watson, *Nature*, **227**, 1029 (1970).
10. Mizutani, S., D. Boettiger, and H. K. Temin, *Nature*, **228**, 424 (1970).
11. Riman, J., and G. S. Beaudreau, *Nature*, **228**, 427 (1970).
12. Spiegelman, S., A. Burny, M. R. Das, J. Keydar, J. Schlom, M. Travnicek, and K. Watson, *Nature*, **228**, 430 (1970).
13. Baltimore, D., and D. Smoler, 3rd Biochemistry-PCRI Winter Symposium, Miami, January 1971 (North-Holland) in press.
14. Vogt, P. K., *Comparative Leukemia Research*, (*1969*) *Bibl. haemat.*, **36**, 153, ed. R. M. Dutcher (Karger, Basel, 1970).
15. Duesberg, P. H., *Proc. Nat. Acad. Sci. USA*, **60**, 1511 (1968).
16. M. Green, M. Rokutanda, K. Fujinaga, C. Gurgo, P. K. Ray, and J. T. Parsons, ed. L. G. Silvestri, 2nd Lepetit Colloquium on *The Biology of Oncogenic Viruses* (North-Holland) p. 193.
17. Kelly, R. R., N. R. Cozzarelli, M. P. Deutscher, I. R. Lehman, and A. J. Kornberg, *Biol. Chem.*, **245**, 39 (1970).
18. Goulian, M., *Proc. Nat. Acad. Sci. USA*, **61**, 284 (1968).
19. Riley, M., B. Maling, and M. I. Chamberlin, *J. Mol. Biol.*, **20**, 359 (1966).
20. Spiegelman, S., A. Burny, M. R. Das, J. Keydar, J. Schlom, M. Travnicek, and K. Watson, *Nature*, **227**, 563 (1970).
21. Duesberg, P. H., *J. Mol. Biol.*, **42**, 485 (1969).
22. Cavalieri, L. F. and E. Carroll, *Nature*, **232**, 254, (1971); Lee Huang, S., and L. F. Cavalieri, *Proc. Nat. Acad. Sci. USA*, **50**, 1116 (1963).

WARREN E. LEVINSON
J. MICHAEL BISHOP
NANCY QUINTRELL
JEAN JACKSON
LOIS FANSHIER

Synthesis of RNA in Normal and Rous Sarcoma Virus-Infected Cells: Effect of Bromodeoxyuridine

Previous efforts to detect virus-specific RNA in cells infected with and transformed by Rous sarcoma virus (RSV) have been unsuccessful (1). This failure may be traced in large measure to the fact that the schemes which have been employed to suppress the background of host RNA synthesis invariably have resulted in suppression of virus production as well. In an effort to achieve selective inhibition of cellular RNA synthesis in RSV-infected cells, we have explored the utility of a number of inhibitors of cell metabolism. This report concerns our experience with one such inhibitor, bromodeoxyuridine (BUDR). In low concentrations, this antimetabolite has a differential effect on normal as opposed to RSV-infected chick embryo fibroblasts, suppressing RNA synthesis in normal cells but having no appreciable effect on that of infected cells. The RNA's extracted from BUDR-inhibited uninfected cells, BUDR-treated infected cells, and untreated cells were examined by electrophoresis in polyacrylamide gels. Neither BUDR nor infection with RSV induced any detectable alteration in the nature of the cellular RNA synthesized, and no virus-specific RNA could be distinguished.

The preparation of chick embryo fibroblast tissue cultures, propagation and assay of RSV [Bryan high titer strain, containing Type 1 Rous-associated virus (RAV-1)], and fixation of cells for microscopic examination were performed as described previously (2). BUDR was purchased from Calbiochem, ^{14}C-uridine (52 mCi/mM) and ^{3}H-uridine (20 Ci/mM) from Schwarz Bio-Research, and ^{14}C-BUDR (19 μCi/mM) from New England Nuclear. Conversion of ^{14}C-uridine into an acid-insoluble state was determined by extracting the cell monolayers with 4% perchloric acid for 1 hour at 4°, then dissolving the residue in 0.3 N NaOH (30

minutes, 60°) and determining the radioactivity in a 0.5-ml aliquot with an end-window counter. RNA was isolated for electrophoretic analysis by dissolving the cell sheets in 0.05 M Na acetate–0.01 M EDTA, pH 5.0, containing 1% sodium dodecyl sulfate, followed by phenol extraction at 60° and ethanol precipitation (3). Electrophoresis was carried out in ethylene diacrylate cross-linked gels of polyacrylamide as described by Bishop et al. (4). Frozen gels were sliced with stacked razor blades (Diversified Scientific Instruments, San Leandro, California), and the slices were hydrolyzed with concentrated NH₄OH and counted in a dioxane scintillation fluid.

The rate of RNA synthesis in uninfected fibroblasts is reduced by 75% after 48 hours in the presence of BUDR (Fig. 1). In contrast, the rate of RNA synthesis in RSV-infected cells is unaffected by exposure to BUDR. Cells infected with RAV-1 alone respond to BUDR in a manner similar to that of uninfected cells. Thus, the resistance to BUDR appears to be induced specifically by the presence of the transforming RSV. Generally, similar results were obtained when the rate of RNA synthesis was estimated by labeling for intervals from 15 minutes to 4 hours.

Three other pertinent variables were examined. First, BUDR reduced the rate of cell growth in both normal and RSV-infected cultures by a factor of two as determined by cell counts on replicate plates. Nevertheless, the cells appeared morphologically normal except for increased fragmentation of nuclei as a consequence of RSV infection (2). Second, the conversation of BUDR into an acid-insoluble state was assessed with ^{14}C-BUDR. RSV-infected cells had uptakes double those of uninfected cells. Therefore, the undiminished rate of RNA synthesis in BUDR-treated infected cells is not attribut-

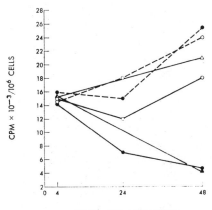

HOURS AFTER ADDING BUDR

FIG. 1. Effect of BUDR on RNA synthesis in normal and infected cells. Chick embryo cells were seeded at a concentration of 1×10^5 cells 35-mm Petri dish. After four hours, the appropriate cultures were infected with either RSV(RAV-1) or RAV-1 at multiplicities of two infectious units per cell. BUDR (15 µg/ml) was added 18 hours later and was present throughout the remainder of the incubation period. At the indicated time points, ^{14}C-uridine was added (0.25 µCi/ml), and incorporation was measured over a 4-hour period. The number of cells on replicate plates was determined for each time point. O——O, uninfected cells without BUDR; ●——●, uninfected cells with BUDR; O---O, RSV-infected cells without BUDR; ●---●, RSV-infected cells with BUDR; △---△, RAV-infected cells without BUDR; ▲——▲, RAV-infected cells with BUDR.

able to simple exclusion of the antimetabolite. Third the effect of BUDR on virus replication was determined. Under the conditions of the experiments illustrated in Fig. 1, no change in virus production was effected by BUDR treatment. However, the same concentration of BUDR, when applied to the cells within the first 12 hours after infection, reduced the 72-hour yield of RSV by a factor of 5. These data resemble the previously reported effect of BUDR on RSV infection (5).

RSV-infected cells have a slightly higher rate of RNA synthesis than do normal, uninfected cells (Fig. 1). This difference has been observed repeatedly in our laboratory

and conforms to previous experience (6–8). It should be noted that the experiments reported here were confined to the first 48 hours following infection, i.e., the period during which the cell population is being actively transformed.

As judged by the results of gel electrophoresis (Fig. 2) neither treatment with BUDR nor infection with RSV has a detectable effect on the nature of the cellular RNA's synthesized. There is no apparent difference between the RNA's synthesized in uninfected and infected cells, in either the presence or the absence of BUDR. This technique did not reveal any RNA which might correspond to the 70S genome of the virus (9). The experiment illustrated in Fig. 2d was designed to detect relatively small quantities of such RNA (the cellular RNA loaded onto the gel contained a total of 275,000 cpm); we do not consider the small deflection of the baseline in the vicinity of the 70S marker to be significant. The viral RNA used as internal marker in this experiment contains five distinct species (70S, 28S, 18S, 7S, and 4S). Purification and analysis of these (particularly the 4S RNA and the previously unrecognized 7S form) will be described in a separate communication (manuscript in preparation). Thus, the data confirm and extend the results of previous experiments in which zonal centrifugation was used in unsuccessful attempts to demonstrate virus-induced RNA's in RSV-infected cells (8).

These data were obtained with 4-hour labeling periods in order to conform to the experiments illustrated in Fig. 1. The RNA species labeled under these conditions are similar to those visible after a steady state label, although traces of ribosomal precursor RNA and some heterogeneous RNA (10) are visible in the gel patterns. We have also examined the RNA labeled by short pulses (5 to 15 minutes) and in pulse-chase experiments designed to elucidate the sequence of events which accompanies the maturation of ribosomal RNA (10). These experiments were performed with zonal centrifugation in sucrose density gradients. They failed to detect any aberration from normal as a consequence of BUDR treatment and/or RSV infection and are not reported in detail.

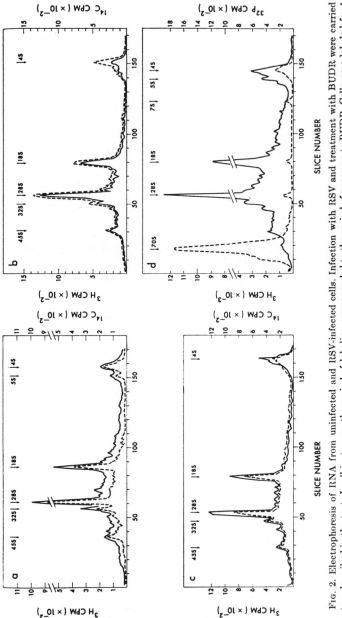

Fig. 2. Electrophoresis of RNA from uninfected and RSV-infected cells. Infection with RSV and treatment with BUDR were carried out as described in the text. In all instances, the period of labeling corresponded to the period of exposure to BUDR. Cells were labeled for 4 hours with ³H-uridine (20 μCi/ ml) or ¹⁴C-uridine (0.25 μCi/ml). RNA was extracted with SDS-phenol and analyzed by electrophoresis in 200-mm gels of 2.25% polyacrylamide. Electrophoresis (5 mμ/gel) was performed at room temperature for 4.75 hours. (a) ³H-RNA from uninfected cells (——) and ¹⁴C-RNA from uninfected cells treated with BUDR (– – –). (b) ³H-RNA from uninfected cells (——) and ¹⁴C-RNA from infected cells (– – –). (c) ³H-RNA from infected cells treated with BUDR (——) and ¹⁴C-RNA from infected cells not treated with BUDR (– – –). (d) ³H-RNA from infected cells treated with BUDR (——) and ³²P-RNA isolated from purified RSV (– – –) virions as described previously (12). The assignment of sedimentation coefficients to the viral RNA species is based on analyses to be presented in a separate communication (manuscript in preparation).

In summary, the preceding data demonstrate the following (1) We have not succeeded in detecting virus-specific RNA in RSV-infected cells, even by the use of the highly sensitive technique of polyacrylamide gel electrophoresis. (2) BUDR at low concentration inhibits the synthesis of RNA in uninfected cells without inducing any apparent quantitative or qualitative abnormalities in the residual RNA synthesis. The mechanism and significance of the latter phenomenon is obscure. The fact that similar results were obtained in various experiments over a tenfold range of uridine concentrations, however, makes it exceedingly unlikely that it simply represents competitive interference with uridine uptake in the presence of BUDR (11).

ACKNOWLEDGMENTS

We would like to thank Dr. Robert Painter for suggesting the use of BUDR to inhibit cellular RNA synthesis. This work was supported by USPHS Grant CA 10223-02, California Division of the American Cancer Society Grant No. 483, and the Cancer Coordinating Committee Grant 2-512501-36240.

REFERENCES

1. ROBINSON, W. S., *In* "The Molecular Biology of Viruses" (J. S. Colter and W. Paranchych, eds), pp. 681–696. Academic Press, New York, 1967.
2. LEVINSON, W. E., *Virology* 32, 74–83 (1967).
3. BISHOP, J. M., and KOCH, G., *J. Biol. Chem.* 242, 1736–1743 (1967).
4. BISHOP, D. H. L., CLAYBROOK, J., and SPIEGELMAN, S., *J. Mol. Biol.* 26, 373-387 (1967).
5. BADER, J., *Virology* 22, 462–468 (1964).
6. GOLDE, A., *Virology* 16, 9–20 (1962).
7. HANAFUSA, H., *Proc. Nat. Acad. Sci. U.S.* 63, 318-325 (1969).
8. COLBY, C., and RUBIN, H., *J. Nat. Cancer Inst.* 43, 437–444 (1969).
9. ROBINSON, W. S., and DUESBERG, P. H., *In* "Molecular Basis of Virology" (H. Fraenkel-Conrat, ed.), pp. 306–331. Rheinhold, New York, 1968.
10. DARNELL, J. E., *Bacteriol Rev.* 32, 262–290 (1968).
11. STECK, T. L., NAKATA, Y., and BADER, J. P., *Biochem. Biophys. Acta* 190, 237–249 (1969).
12. ROBINSON, W. S., PITKANEN, A., and RUBIN, H., *Proc. Nat. Acad. Sci. U.S.* 54, 137–144 (1965).

RNA-dependent DNA Polymerase in Virions of Rous Sarcoma Virus

HOWARD M. TEMIN
SATOSHI MIZUTANI

INFECTION of sensitive cells by RNA sarcoma viruses requires the synthesis of new DNA different from that synthesized in the S-phase of the cell cycle (refs. 1, 2 and unpublished results of D. Boettiger and H. M. T.); production of RNA tumour viruses is sensitive to actinomycin D[3,4]; and cells transformed by RNA tumour viruses have new DNA which hybridizes with viral RNA[5,6]. These are the basic observations essential to the DNA provirus hypothesis—replication of RNA tumour viruses takes place through a DNA intermediate, not through an RNA intermediate as does the replication of other RNA viruses[7].

Formation of the provirus is normal in stationary chicken cells exposed to Rous sarcoma virus (RSV), even in the presence of 0·5 µg/ml. cycloheximide (our unpublished results). This finding, together with the discovery of polymerases in virions of vaccinia virus and of reovirus[8-11], suggested that an enzyme that would synthesize DNA from an RNA template might be present in virions of RSV. We now report data supporting the existence of such an enzyme, and we learn that David Baltimore has independently discovered a similar enzyme in virions of Rauscher leukaemia virus[12].

This work was supported by a US Public Health Service research grant from the National Cancer Institute. H. M. T. holds a research career development award from the National Cancer Institute.

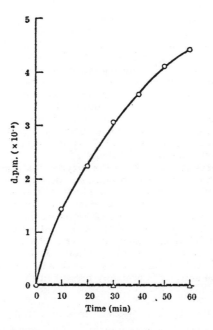

Fig. 1. Kinetics of incorporation. Virus treated with 'Nonidet' and dithiothreitol at 0° C and incubated at 37° C (O—O) or 80° C (△ - - - △) for 10 min was assayed in a standard polymerase assay. O, Unheated; △, heated.

The sources of virus and methods of concentration have been described[13]. All preparations were carried out in sterile conditions. Concentrated virus was placed on a layer of 15 per cent sucrose and centrifuged at 25,000 r.p.m. for 1 h in the 'SW 25.1' rotor of the Spinco ultracentrifuge on to a cushion of 60 per cent sucrose. The virus band was collected from the interphase and further purified by equilibrium sucrose density gradient centrifugation[14]. Virus further purified by sucrose velocity density gradient centrifugation gave the same results.

Table 1. ACTIVATION OF ENZYME

System	^{3}H-TTP incorporated (d.p.m.)
No virions	0
Non-disrupted virions	255
Virions disrupted with 'Nonidet'	
At 0° + DTT	6,730
At 0° − DTT	4,420
At 40° + DTT	5,000
At 40° − DTT	425

Purified virions untreated or incubated for 5 min at 0° C or 40° C with 0.25 per cent 'Nonidet P-40' (Shell Chemical Co.) with 0 or 1 per cent dithiothreitol (DTT) (Sigma) were assayed in the standard polymerase assay.

The polymerase assay consisted of 0·125 μmoles each of dATP, dCTP, and dGTP (Calbiochem) (in 0·02 M Tris-HCl buffer at pH 8·0, containing 0·33 M EDTA and 1·7 mM 2-mercaptoethanol); 1·25 μmoles of MgCl$_2$ and 2·5 μmoles of KCl; 2·5 μg phosphoenolpyruvate (Calbiochem); 10 μg pyruvate kinase (Calbiochem); 2·5 μCi of ^{3}H-TTP (Schwarz) (12 Ci/mmole); and 0·025 ml. of enzyme (10^8 focus forming units of disrupted Schmidt-Ruppin virus, $A_{280\ nm} = 0·30$) in a total volume of 0·125 ml. Incubation was at 40° C for 1 h. 0·025 ml. of the reaction mixture was withdrawn and assayed for acid-insoluble counts by the method of Furlong[15].

To observe full activity of the enzyme, it was necessary to treat the virions with a non-ionic detergent (Tables 1 and 4). If the treatment was at 40° C the presence of dithiothreitol (DTT) was necessary to recover activity. In most preparations of virions, however, there was some activity: 5–20 per cent of the disrupted virions, in the absence of detergent treatment, which probably represents disrupted virions in the preparation. It is known that virions of RNA tumour viruses are easily disrupted[16,17], so that the activity is probably present in the nucleoid of the virion.

Table 2. REQUIREMENTS FOR ENZYME ACTIVITY

System	^{3}H-TTP incorporated (d.p.m.)
Complete	5,675
Without MgCl$_2$	186
Without MgCl$_2$, with MnCl$_2$	5,570
Without MgCl$_2$, with CaCl$_2$	18
Without dATP	897
Without dCTP	1,780
Without dGTP	2,190

Virus treated with 'Nonidet' and dithiothreitol at 0° C was incubated in the standard polymerase assay with the substitutions listed.

The kinetics of incorporation with disrupted virions are shown in Fig. 1. Incorporation is rapid for 1 h. Other experiments show that incorporation continues at about the same rate for the second hour. Preheating disrupted virus at 80° C prevents any incorporation, and so does pretreatment of disrupted virus with crystalline trypsin.

Fig. 2 demonstrates that there is an absolute requirement for MgCl$_2$, 10 mM being the optimum concentration. The data in Table 2 show that MnCl$_2$ can substitute for MgCl$_2$ in the polymerase assay, but CaCl$_2$ cannot. Other experiments show that a monovalent cation is not required for activity, although 20 mM KCl causes a 15 per

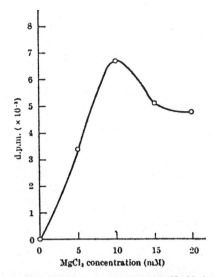

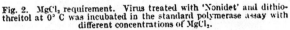

Fig. 2. MgCl₂ requirement. Virus treated with 'Nonidet' and dithiothreitol at 0° C was incubated in the standard polymerase assay with different concentrations of MgCl₂.

cent stimulation. Higher concentrations of KCl are inhibitory: 60 per cent inhibition was observed at 80 mM.

When the amount of disrupted virions present in the polymerase assay was varied, the amount of incorporation varied with second-order kinetics. When incubation was carried out at different temperatures, a broad optimum between 40° C and 50° C was found. (The high temperature of this optimum may relate to the fact that the normal host of the virus is the chicken.) When incubation was carried out at different pHs, a broad optimum at pH 8–9·5 was found.

Table 2 demonstrates that all four deoxyribonucleotide triphosphates are required for full activity, but some activity was present when only three deoxyribonucleotide triphosphates were added and 10–20 per cent of full activity was still present with only two deoxyribonucleotide triphosphates. The activity in the presence of three deoxyribonucleotide triphosphates is probably the result of the presence of deoxyribonucleotide triphosphates in the virion. Other host components are known to be incorporated in the virion of RNA tumour viruses[18,19].

Table 3. RNA DEPENDENCE OF POLYMERASE ACTIVITY

Treatment	³H-TTP incorporated (d.p.m.)
Non-treated disrupted virions	9,110
Disrupted virions preincubated with ribonuclease A (50 µg/ml.) at 20° C for 1 h	2,650
Disrupted virions preincubated with ribonuclease A (1 mg/ml.) at 0° C for 1 h	137
Disrupted virions preincubated with lysozyme (50 µg/ml.) at 0° C for 1 h	9,650

Disrupted virions were incubated with ribonuclease A (Worthington) which was heated at 80° C for 10 min, or with lysozyme at the indicated concentration in the specified conditions, and a standard polymerase assay was performed.

The data in Table 3 demonstrate that incorporation of thymidine triphosphate was more than 99 per cent abolished if the virions were pretreated at 0° with 1 mg ribonuclease per ml. Treatment with 50 μg/ml. ribonuclease at 20° C did not prevent all incorporation of thymidine triphosphate, which suggests that the RNA of the virion may be masked by protein. (Lysozyme was added as a control for non-specific binding of ribonuclease to DNA.) Because the ribonuclease was heated for 10 min at 80° C or 100° C before use to destroy deoxyribonuclease it seems that intact RNA is necessary for incorporation of thymidine triphosphate.

Table 4. SOURCE OF POLYMERASE

Source	³H-TTP incorporated (d.p.m.)
Virions of SRV	1,410
Disrupted virions of SRV	5,675
Virions of AMV	1,875
Disrupted virions of AMV	12,850
Disrupted pellet from supernatant of uninfected cells	0

Virions of Schmidt-Ruppin virus (SRV) were prepared as before (experiment of Table 2). Virions of avian myeloblastosis virus (AMV) and a pellet from uninfected cells were prepared by differential centrifugation. All disrupted preparations were treated with 'Nonidet' and dithiothreitol at 0° C and assayed in a standard polymerase assay. The material used per tube was originally from 45 ml. of culture fluid for SRV, 20 ml. for AMV, and 20 ml. for uninfected cells.

To determine whether the enzyme is present in supernatants of normal cells or in RNA leukaemia viruses, the experiment of Table 4 was performed. Normal cell supernatant did not contain activity even after treatment with 'Nonidet'. Virions of avian myeloblastosis virus (AMV) contained activity that was increased ten-fold by treatment with 'Nonidet'.

The nature of the product of the polymerase assay was investigated by treating portions with deoxyribonuclease, ribonuclease or KOH. About 80 per cent of the product was made acid soluble by treatment with deoxyribonuclease, and the product was resistant to ribonuclease and KOH (Table 5).

Table 5. NATURE OF PRODUCT

Treatment	Residual acid-insoluble ³H-TTP (d.p.m.)	
	Experiment A	Experiment B
Buffer	10,200	8,350
Deoxyribonuclease	697	1,520
Ribonuclease	10,900	7,200
KOH	—	8,250

A standard polymerase assay was performed with 'Nonidet' treated virions. The product was incubated in buffer or 0·3 M KOH at 37° C for 20 h or with (A) 1 mg/ml. or (B) 50 μg/ml. of deoxyribonuclease I (Worthington), or with 1 mg/ml. of ribonuclease A (Worthington) for 1 h at 37° C. and portions were removed and tested for acid-insoluble counts.

To determine if the polymerase might also make RNA, disrupted virions were incubated with the four ribonucleotide triphosphates, including ³H-UTP (Schwarz, 3·2 Ci/mmole). With either MgCl₂ or MnCl₂ in the incu-

30

bation mixture, no incorporation was detected. In a parallel incubation with deoxyribonucleotide triphosphates, 12,200 d.p.m. of ^{3}H-TTP was incorporated.

These results demonstrate that there is a new polymerase inside the virions of RNA tumour viruses. It is not present in supernatants of normal cells but is present in virions of avian sarcoma and leukaemia RNA tumour viruses. The polymerase seems to catalyse the incorporation of deoxyribonucleotide triphosphates into DNA from an RNA template. Work is being performed to characterize further the reaction and the product. If the present results and Baltimore's results[12] with Rauscher leukaemia virus are upheld, they will constitute strong evidence that the DNA provirus hypothesis is correct and that RNA tumour viruses have a DNA genome when they are in cells and an RNA genome when they are in virions. This result would have strong implications for theories of viral carcinogenesis and, possibly, for theories of information transfer in other biological systems[20].

This work was supported by a US Public Health Service research grant from the National Cancer Institute. H. M. T. holds a research career development award from the National Cancer Institute.

[1] Temin, H. M., *Cancer Res.*, **28**, 1835 (1968).
[2] Murray, R. K., and Temin, H. M., *Intern. J. Cancer* (in the press).
[3] Temin, H. M., *Virology*, **20**, 577 (1963).
[4] Baluda, M. B., and Nayak, D. P., *J. Virol.*, **4**, 554 (1969).
[5] Temin, H. M., *Proc. US Nat. Acad. Sci.*, **52**, 323 (1964).
[6] Baluda, M. B., and Nayak, D. P., in *Biology of Large RNA Viruses* (edit. by Barry, R., and Mahy, B.) (Academic Press, London, 1970).
[7] Temin, H. M., *Nat. Cancer Inst. Monog.*, **17**, 557 (1964).
[8] Kates, J. R., and McAuslan, B. R., *Proc. US Nat. Acad. Sci.*, **57**, 314 (1967).
[9] Munyon, W., Paoletti, E., and Grace, J. T., *Proc. US Nat. Acad. Sci.*, **58**, 2280 (1967).
[10] Borsa, J., and Graham, A. F., *Biochem. Biophys. Res. Commun.*, **33**, 895 (1968).
[11] Sharkin, A. J., and Sipe, J. D., *Proc. US Nat. Acad. Sci.*, **61**, 1462 (1968).
[12] Baltimore, D., *Nature*, **226**, 1209 (1970) (preceding article).
[13] Altaner, C., and Temin, H. M., *Virology*, **40**, 118 (1970).
[14] Robinson, W. S., Pitkanen, A., and Rubin, H., *Proc. US Nat. Acad. Sci.*, **54**, 137 (1965).
[15] Furlong, N. B., *Meth. Cancer Res.*, **3**, 27 (1967).
[16] Vogt, P. K., *Adv. Virus. Res.*, **11**, 293 (1965).
[17] Bauer, H., and Schafer, W., *Virology*, **29**, 494 (1966).
[18] Bauer, H., *Z. Naturforsch.*, **21b**, 453 (1966).
[19] Erikson, R. L., *Virology*, **37**, 124 (1969).
[20] Temin, H. M., *Persp. Biol. Med.* (in the press).

Synthesis of the RNA of RNA-Containing Tumor Viruses

JOHN P. BADER

INTRODUCTION

The RNA-containing oncogenic viruses are unique among viruses in morphological, antigenic, and biochemical characteristics, as well as in their biological effects on the infected organism (and cell), and in their biochemical requirements for infection. Despite group, species, and strain differences, certain features of virion structure and virus production obtain without exception. These include physical characteristics of the RNA and biochemical requirements for infection.

These tumorigenic viruses all contain RNAs of presumptive high molecular weight (about 10^7 daltons) (Robinson *et al.*, 1965; Harel *et al.*, 1965; Duesberg and Blair, 1966; Valentine and Bader, 1968), which have been reported recently to undergo molecular changes during treatment with heat or dimethyl sulfoxide (Duesberg, 1968; Blair and Duesberg, 1968; Duesberg and Cardiff, 1968; Erickson, 1969). Studies on the structure of viral RNA (vRNA) require virus of exceptional integrity. The rapid thermal inactivation rate of infectivity demands that virus be sequestered soon after

production. The investigations reported here analyze virus production through the labeling of viral RNA, and in a separate paper a characterization of the vRNA is presented (Bader and Steck, 1969).

Synthesis of DNA during the early stages of infection is required for successful infection by avian and murine tumor viruses (Bader, 1964, 1965a, b, 1966a; Nakata and Bader, 1968), and continuous transcription of DNA into RNA in later stages is necessary for virus production (Temin, 1963; Bader, 1964, 1966b; Bases and King, 1967). The viruses are simultaneously completed and released from infected cells by a process of budding from the plasma membrane. The minimum interval reported between initial infection by Rous sarcoma virus and the appearance of progeny virus was 8 hours (Bader, 1966a; Hanafusa and Hanafusa, 1966). This was also the approximate interval measured for the requisite DNA synthesis. Minimal time intervals for the essential DNA synthetic period probably could be obtained using synchronized cell cultures, but such studies have not yet been reported.

The interval between synthesis of viral RNA and the release of virus has not previously been examined. The experiments presented here were addressed to the kinetics of transfer of viral RNA from the site of synthesis to the completed virion.

The performance of such a series of experiments required a uniformity of cellular metabolism and virus production from one experiment to another. Although reasonable results were obtained using virus productive Rous sarcoma virus (RSV)-infected cells, a serial line of cells producing murine leukemia virus (MLV), the JLSV₅ line, was found more favorable for critical analyses. The synthesis and detection of RSV and MLV RNAs are described.

MATERIALS AND METHODS

Virus-producing cells. Cell cultures were grown as monolayers in 10-cm plastic petri dishes, using a humidified CO_2 atmosphere incubator set at 37°. Chick embryo cells were trypsinized and grown 3 days as primary cultures in Eagle's minimal essential medium (MEM) containing 10% calf serum and 10% tryptose phosphate broth (Difco). Secondary cultures were exposed to Rous sarcoma virus–Rous associated virus₁ (RSV-RAV₁, 1 focus-forming unit per cell) and then cultivated in medium in which calf serum was replaced by fetal bovine serum. After two subsequent transfers at 3-day intervals, cultures were used in labeling experiments. Mouse splenic cells (JLSV₅) producing murine leukemia virus (MLV, Rauscher) were cultivated in a growth medium (GM) containing 5% fetal bovine serum and MEM. Labeling experiments were done on the day after culture transfer of both cell lines.

Radioactive labeling of vRNA. Uridine-5-³H (50 μCi/ml, 5–25 Ci/mmole) was added in 3 ml of MEM containing 5% fetal bovine serum to cultures. Except where stated, the radioactive label was removed after 15 min incubation at 37°, cultures were rinsed four times with warm MEM, and 3 ml of GM was added. Fluids were later removed, centrifuged at 3000 g to remove floating cells, and the supernatants were frozen at −70° until assayed, usually within 24 hours.

Analysis of vRNA. Initial experiments utilized sucrose gradients as described previously (Valentine and Bader, 1968). Virus was purified by ammonium sulfate precipitation and density banding in 15–55% gradients. The RNA was extracted using 1% sodium lauryl sulfate (SLS), carrier yeast RNA (1 mg/sample), pronase (50 μg/ml), and phenol. After precipitation from the aqueous layer with sodium acetate (2%) and ethanol (2 vol), the RNA was sedimented through a 5–20% sucrose gradient for 2 hours at 105,000 g. RNA from both RSV-RAV₁ and MLV presented radioactive peaks with sedimentation constant about 70 S. The RNA from this region was precipitated with sodium acetate and ethanol and the pellet resuspended in "electrophoresis buffer."

In experiments involving rapid labeling and extraction, culture fluids were subjected to centrifugation at 100,000 g for 2 hours in the Spinco No. 40 Rotor. The resulting pellet was exposed to 1% SLS in "electrophoresis buffer" after adding polyvinyl sulfate (PVS, 50 μg/ml).

Electrophoresis in polyacrylamide gels. Resolution of RNA was made by electrophoresis in slab gels as described by Peacock and Dingman (1967). Gel mixtures contained 1.9% acrylamide, 0.1% N,N'-methylenebisacrylamide, 0.5% agarose, and 0.1% SLS. Ammonium persulfate (0.05%) and dimethylaminopropionitrile (0.4%) were added to catalyze polymerization. The slab gels were prepared to contain 8–12 samples per gel, facilitating comparative analysis of migration velocities. "Electrophoresis buffer" contained Tris-HCl (0.09 M), boric acid (0.09 M), and Na₂EDTA (0.0025 M). Gels were run at 12°, 200 V (11 V/cm), 50 mA, for 1 hour in preliminary experiments, for 1.5 hours subsequently.

Each sample track was cut into 1-mm sections, which were exposed overnight to 0.1 ml NaOH (0.3 M) to hydrolyze the RNA. One milliliter of NCS reagent (Nuclear Chicago Corp.) was added and samples counted in 25:1 toluene–Liquifluor (New England Nuclear Corp.) in a Packard scintillation counter.

Cytoplasmic RNA extracted from rat

embryo cells in culture served as standards. After electrophoresis, gel strips containing RNA standards were rinsed in H_2O, then exposed to methylene blue (0.002% in 0.01 M acetic acid) overnight. Stained bands regularly were found at regions expected for 28 S and 18 S ribosomal RNA. Occasionally cellular DNA also was included as a standard.

Labeling of cellular components. Synthesis of cellular RNA was monitored by exposure of cells to uridine-5-^{3}H (3 μCi in 3 ml) and measuring the incorporation into trichloroacetic acid-insoluble material. Protein synthesis was analyzed by the incorporation of ^{14}C amino acids (3 μCi in 3 ml) into acid-insoluble material.

Nuclei and cytoplasm were separated by exposing the cellular monolayers to the detergent Nonidet P-40 (0.5% in Tris-dextrose buffer containing 2 mM $MgCl_2$) for 10 min. Centrifugation for 10 min at 3000 g sedimented the nuclei. Prior labeling of cellular DNA with thymidine-^{3}H demonstrated that less than 1% of the DNA was found in the cytoplasmic supernatant by this fractionation.

Antimetabolites. To test the efficacy of antimetabolites on the metabolism of JLSV$_5$ cells, various dilutions of the compounds were added for 1 hour. Radioactive precursor was then added, and incorporation during the subsequent hour into perchloric acid-insoluble material was determined. Actinomycin D (2 μg/ml) reduced the incorporation of uridine-^{3}H into RNA by 99%; cycloheximide (10 μg/ml) or puromycin (50 μg/ml) reduced the incorporation into protein by 99%; cytosine arabinoside (1-β-D-arabinofuranosylcytosine, 10^{-4} M) reduced DNA synthesis by 95%; 2,6-diaminopurine riboside (10^{-4} M) reduced RNA synthesis by less than 20%.

RESULTS

Detection of Viral RNA

The analysis of production of RNA required first a quantitative system for detection of the specific RNA. Large molecular weight vRNA could be easily separated from cellular RNAs by velocity sedimentation in sucrose gradients (Valentine and Bader,

1968). However, such zonal centrifugation as an analytical method lacked resolution, reproducibility, and convenience. Polyacrylamide-agarose gels have been used in the electrophoretic analysis of cellular RNAs (Peacock and Dingman, 1967, 1968), and the migration of vRNAs in a polyacrylamide-agarose gel mixture was analyzed. Phenol-extracted vRNAs from both RSV-RAV$_1$ and MLV migrated at rates compatible with the projected estimate for RNA of molecular weight about 10^7 (Fig. 1). The radioactivity appeared in bands distinct from those of dominant cellular nucleic acids, 45 S RNA, DNA, ribosomal RNA (28 S, 18 S), etc.

Considerable time was required usually in the SLS-phenol extraction of vRNA from virions, and quantitative recoveries after precipitation of the RNA with ethanol were variable. It was found that addition of SLS to either RSV or MLV was sufficient to release the vRNA. Direct application of SLS-treated virions to the gels resulted in complete recovery of radioactive vRNA in the expected zone (Fig. 1).

The radioactive material obtained by SLS treatment was shown in fact to be RNA. Addition of ribonuclease to the viral pellets exposed to SLS resulted in the disappearance of radioactivity from the vRNA region (Fig. 1). Since SLS itself was found to be ineffective in preventing the enzymatic degradation of RNA, polyvinyl sulfate was included subsequently in the SLS solution as a prophylactic against ribonuclease.

Purification of the viruses by isopycnic banding in sucrose gradients was time consuming. Earlier experiments involving concentration of virus by pelleting resulted in considerable loss of virus infectivity; nondissociable virus aggregation presumably occurred. Since aggregation was unlikely to affect the molecular configuration of vRNA, and the anticipated investigations did not involve infectivity measurements, the concentration of virus by simple pelleting by high-speed centrifugation was investigated.

The pattern of RNA labeling of cell culture fluids was examined at various intervals after exposure of cells to uridine-^{3}H. Culture fluids collected at hourly intervals for 5

34

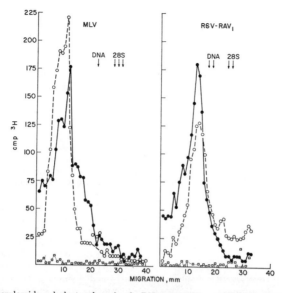

Fig. 1. Polyacrylamide gel electrophoresis of vRNA of MLV or RSV-RAV₁. Virions labeled with uridine-³H were purified by density banding in 15–55% sucrose gradients. RNA was extracted with phenol (○) and the electrophoretic migration compared with that of unextracted virions exposed only to SLS (●). MLV and RSV-RAV₁ were analyzed in separate experiments. SLS-treated virions were also exposed to ribonuclease (□) before gel analysis. Arrows indicate the position of marker nucleic acids.

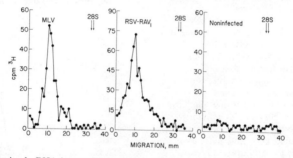

Fig. 2. Analysis of vRNA from pelleted virions after short labeling periods. Cells were exposed to uridine-³H (300 μCi in 3 ml) for 15 min, rinsed, and incubated at 37°. Virus collected at hourly intervals for 5 hours was pooled and sedimented at 105,000 g, exposed to PVS (50 μg/ml) then SLS (1%) and added directly to polyacrylamide gels. Culture fluids from uninfected chick embryo cells were similarly analyzed.

hours after uridine-³H contained significant radioactivity only in the vRNA region, provided floating cells were removed before ultracentrifugation (Fig. 2). No significant radioactivity was found in regions of DNA, 28 S, 18 S, 5 S, or 4 S cellular RNAs during this time (see Bader and Steck, 1969). Culture fluids collected at the same time from uninfected chick embryo cells revealed no significant radioactivity in the vRNA region

35

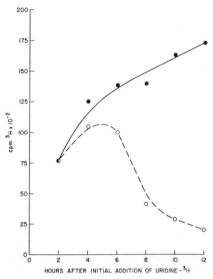

FIG. 3. Uridine-³H labeling of virion RNA. Uridine-³H (300 μCi in 3 ml) was added to JLSV₅ cells for 2 hours and replaced with uridine-³H containing medium (●) or GM (○) at 2-hour intervals. Radioactivity in the vRNA of sedimented virions was determined by exposure of virions to SLS and subsequent electrophoresis.

(Fig. 2). Labeled cellular RNA appeared in culture fluids increasingly after 5 hours, presumably owing to the inadvertent occasional lysis of labeled cells.

It was possible then to analyze the release of vRNA after short labeling periods by pelleting the virions, rupturing the virions with SLS in the presence of polyvinyl sulfate, subjecting the lysate to electrophoresis in polyacrylamide gels, and measuring the radioactivity in the appropriate area.

Uridine-³H Labeling of Virions

Several procedures for the labeling of MLV were designed to determine a time course for synthesis and release of vRNA: (a) Uridine-³H was added to JLSV₅ cells and replenished at 2-hour intervals. It was possible that a single short labeling period would be insufficient to adequately label the vRNA to be extruded, and thus repeated exposures were given (Fig. 3). (b) Uridine-³H

was added to cells and removed 2 hours later, the cultures were rinsed, and growth medium was replaced then and at 2-hour intervals (Fig. 3). In both cases labeled vRNA was found in the culture fluids of the first medium change, indicating that 2 hours was a sufficient interval between the completion of synthesis of vRNA and its incorporation into virions. (c) In a subsequent experiment, uridine-³H was added for 15 min, removed, the cultures were rinsed, and growth medium added and replaced at hourly intervals. Analysis of the hourly harvests (Fig. 4) showed no detectable radioactive vRNA in samples prior to the 2-hour sample but significant amounts thereafter.

Cultures continuously exposed to uridine-³H produced labeled vRNA in increasing amounts over the 12-hour period, although the rate of increase diminished with time (Fig. 3). When label was removed at 2 hours, the maximum amount of vRNA-³H was found 4 hours later. In various other experiments using shorter labeling periods, and hourly collections, vRNA was found maximally labeled within 5 hours after removal of radioactive uridine (Fig. 4). However, the increase in rate of synthesis after the initial 2 hours was relatively

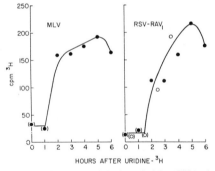

FIG. 4. Uridine-³H labeling of virion RNA of MLV and RSV-RAV₁. Uridine-³H (150 μCi in 3 ml) was added to cells for 15 min then replaced with GM. At various intervals fluids were collected and replaced. The radioactivity in the vRNA of pelleted virus was determined. The results of two experiments on RSV-RAV₁ collections at different time intervals are shown. Points in parentheses represent background counts evenly distributed in the vRNA region.

36

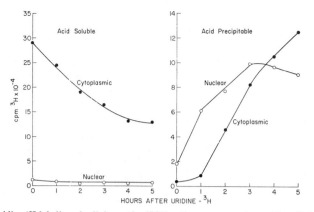

HOURS AFTER URIDINE - ^{3}H

Fig. 5. Uridine-^{3}H labeling of cellular pools. JLSV$_5$ cells were exposed to uridine-^{3}H (3 μCi in 3 ml) for 15 min, then rinsed. At hourly intervals cells were separated into nuclear and cytoplasmic fractions, and TCA-soluble and -insoluble radioactivity was analyzed.

minor, indicating that maximal rates had essentially been reached by 2 hours. Despite maximum labeling of vRNA by 5 hours after removal of uridine-^{3}H, incorporation of radioactive vRNA into virions continued for several hours thereafter.

The labeling of the RNA of RSV-RAV$_1$ (Fig. 4) followed essentially the same time course as the MLV. No significant radioactivity was found in the RNA of virions before 2 hours, and maximum labeling was found within 5 hours after removing label. However, inconsistencies in the labeling of RSV-RAV$_1$ after the initial delay prevented confident assessments and experiments with this virus were discontinued.

Labeling of Cellular Pools.

The time course of incorporation of uridine-^{3}H into nuclear and cytoplasmic RNA of JLSV$_5$ cells was analyzed to aid in the interpretation of virus labeling experiments. Although the acid-soluble radioactivity, representing nucleic acid precursors, decreased steadily after removal of uridine-^{3}H from the medium, over one-third of the original radioactivity could still be found in this fraction after 5 hours' incubation (Fig. 5). This high residual pool of precursors explains the continuous labeling of virions long after label is removed from the medium.

Nuclear RNA is rapidly labeled and radioactivity increases, reaching a maximum at 3 hours (Fig. 5). As in other systems, a lag in the labeling of cytoplasmic RNA was observed. By comparing the total number of counts per minute of uridine-^{3}H incorporated into cellular RNA with those incorporated into virion RNA during 1 hour, it could be calculated that 1–10 counts are incorporated into the virion RNA of MLV for every 10^5 in cellular RNA of JLSV$_5$ cells.

The Minimum Interval

Determination of the minimum interval between labeling and envelopment of MLV-vRNA required a closer examination of the period between 1 and 2 hours. One group of JLSV$_5$ cultures was continuously exposed to uridine-^{3}H. Label was removed from a second group to determine whether possible differences in the pool of radioactive precursors would affect the kinetics of labeling of vRNA. Label appeared in virion RNA of the 80-min sample but not earlier (Fig. 6). Other unpublished experiments revealed that labeling of JLSV$_5$ cellular RNA occurs within 5 min after addition of uridine-^{3}H, indicating that processing of exogenous uridine-^{3}H to intracellular uridine-^{3}H triphosphate occurs within this interval. Therefore, the minimum interval between the labeling of vRNA and its appearance in virions is

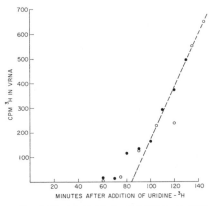

FIG. 6. The interval between labeling of vRNA and appearance in virions. Uridine-³H was added to JLSV₅ cultures and removed from one group (O) after 1 hour and replaced with GM. The second group (●) was exposed continuously to label. Fluids were collected at 10- or 15-min intervals and processed for determination of radioactive vRNA.

heximide and puromycin, also prevented the extrusion of labeled vRNA when added immediately after exposure of cells to uridine-³H (Table 1). In these three cases only, the recorded radioactivity had a heterogeneous distribution rather than distinctive peaks in the vRNA region.

Inhibition of DNA synthesis by cytosine arabinoside had no significant effect on the appearance of vRNA, consistent with its failure to prevent Rous sarcoma virus production when added during late stages of the productive cycle (Bader, 1966a).

Apparently 2,6-diaminopurine riboside can be incorporated into RNA, rendering that RNA defective, and in this manner inhibits the production of infectious Rous sarcoma virus (Bader, 1966a). In the present system the diaminopurine had no inhibitory effect on the release of vRNA during the first 2-hour period (Table 1), but inhibition was noted an hour later. It is likely that the continued production of MLV-RNA depends upon functional cellular RNA, as was indi-

concluded to be 70–75 min. The rate of release of radioactive vRNA increased after its initial appearance. After 20 min a nearly constant rate was found in cultures continuously or temporarily exposed to uridine-³H.

Effect of Metabolic Inhibitors

Previous studies demonstrated an inhibitory effect of certain antimetabolites on the production of Rous sarcoma virus (Bader, 1964, 1966a). Sampling at 4-hour intervals suggested that antagonists of RNA or protein synthesis rapidly prevented the further production of infectious virus, while virus growth continued during inhibition of DNA synthesis. The effect of various antimetabolites on the appearance of MLV-RNA extracellularly was examined. In this experiment, antimetabolites were added immediately after a 15-min exposure of cells to uridine-³H. Culture fluids were collected 2 and 3 hours later.

Actinomycin D, which prevents transcription of DNA, inhibited the appearance of extracellular vRNA as determined by the failure to detect labeled vRNA (Table 1). Two inhibitors of protein synthesis, cyclo-

TABLE 1

EFFECT OF ANTIMETABOLITES ON THE APPEARANCE OF RADIOACTIVE vRNA IN VIRIONS[a]

Antimetabolite	Hours after uridine-³H pulse	
	2	3
None	208	215
Actinomycin D	(39)	(14)
Cycloheximide	(76)	(20)
Puromycin	(19)	(30)
Cytosine arabinoside	192	111
2,6-Diaminopurine riboside	333	54

[a] JLSV₅ cells were exposed to 300 μCi of uridine-³H in 3 ml of growth medium (GM). Fifteen minutes later the radioactive fluids were removed, the cultures were washed, and GM containing antimetabolites was added. Fluids were collected and replaced with antimetabolite media 2 hours later, and these fluids were collected the next hour. RNA in sedimented virus (Materials and Methods) was analyzed by electrophoresis in polyacrylamide gels, and radioactivity appearing in the area expected of vRNA was determined. Numbers in parentheses were found in a broad heterogeneous distribution, rather than in the peak characteristic of vRNA.

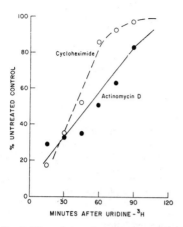

FIG. 7. Effect of time of addition of actionmycin D and cycloheximide on the extracellular appearance of vRNA. JLSV₅ cells were exposed to uridine -³H (150 μCi in 3 ml) for 15 min, then rinsed, and GM was added. At 15-min intervals thereafter, actinomycin D (2 μg/ml) or cycloheximide (10 μg/ml) was added. Two hours after the labeling period, culture fluids were collected and the radioactivity in vRNA of pelleted virus was determined.

cated by previous studies on RSV (Bader, 1966b).

The Delayed Addition of Antimetabolites

If actinomycin D or cycloheximide were only preventing the synthesis of virus constituents, then the delayed addition of antimetabolites after labeling should allow the eventual release of synthesized radioactive vRNA. On the other hand, inhibition of completion of virions by actinomycin D or cycloheximide would be apparent in a complete subsequent suppression of labeled extracellular vRNA. The effect of actinomycin D and cycloheximide added at various times between initial exposure to uridine-³H and the appearance of labeled virus was examined. Culture fluids were removed for assay of vRNA 2 hours after labeling. Some radioactive vRNA was released when as little as 15 min elapsed between the radioactive pulse and the addition of actinomycin D (Fig. 7). Indeed, at 1 hour when no labeled virus had yet been released, about

50% of the vRNA was destined to appear in virions in the presence of actinomycin D. The data demonstrate that vRNA which has been completed intracellularly can make its way into virions in the presence of actinomycin D.

Cycloheximide is ineffective in preventing the extrusion of RNA-labeled virions if added 1 hour or later after uridine-³H (Fig. 7), and significant radioactive vRNA appears if after the uridine-³H pulse a delay of 15 min is allowed before the addition of cycloheximide.

The effect of actinomycin D or cycloheximide on the continued production of radioactive virus after virion ³H-RNA had begun to appear in the medium was also examined. A 2-hour interval after labeling was allowed before the antimetabolites were added. Production of radioactive virus continued during the first hour and then dropped sharply (Fig. 8). The results demonstrate again that virus completion occurs under conditions that limit RNA or protein synthesis. Failure to continue producing labeled virus can be attributed to an inhibi-

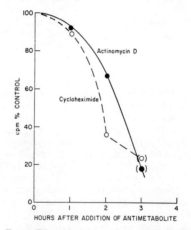

FIG. 8. Effect of actinomycin D and cycloheximide on the continued production of virion RNA. Uridine-³H (150 μCi in 3 ml) was added to JLSV₅ cells for 15 min, then replaced with GM. Two hours later, and at hourly intervals, culture fluids were replaced with actinomycin D (2 μg/ml) or cycloheximide (10 μg/ml) containing GM. The collected fluids were analyzed for radioactivity in vRNA.

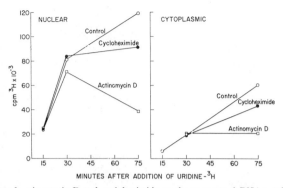

FIG. 9. Effects of actinomycin D and cycloheximide on the progress of RNA synthesis. JLSV₅ cells were exposed to uridine-³H for 15 min, then rinsed. Actinomycin D (2 μg/ml) or cycloheximide (10 μg/ml) was added. At the various indicated times cells were separated into nuclear and cytoplasmic fractions and the amount of radioactivity in TCA-precipitable material was determined.

tion either of synthesis of virus components or of other critical materials.

Effects of Actinomycin D and Cycloheximide on Metabolism

To interpret the activities of actinomycin D (2 μg/ml) and cycloheximide (10 μg/ml) on vRNA release, their effects on cellular metabolism were examined. The imposition of actinomycin D or cycloheximide on JLSV₅ cells induced no recognizable morphological changes for several hours beyond the above experimental periods. Although the action of actinomycin D was irreversible, cell growth resumed after removal of cycloheximide.

Inhibition of cellular protein synthesis was observed within 15 min when cycloheximide and leucine-¹⁴C were added simultaneously, and labeling of protein was reduced to less than 20% of the controls within 30 min of cycloheximide addition. Therefore, conditions which inhibited protein synthesis failed to prevent virus completion; release of virus was not dependent upon simultaneous protein synthesis. Actinomycin D had no detectable effect on leucine-¹⁴C incorporation during the first 15 min, and less than 50% decrease was noted by the end of 1 hour.

Effects on the progress of RNA synthesis were also examined. Simultaneous addition of cycloheximide with uridine-³H produced

no effect on the incorporation of label into RNA during the first 15 min, although extension of the interval to 1 hour gave significant inhibition. Actinomycin D decreased RNA synthesis within 15 min.

When actinomycin D was added to cells after a prior 15-min exposure to uridine-³H, RNA labeling continued for 15 min in both nuclear and cytoplasmic fractions (Fig. 9). Extension to 1 hour revealed that actinomycin D prevented further accumulation of label in the cytoplasm, and that label was lost from nuclear RNA.

Increases in incorporation of uridine-³H into both nuclear and cytoplasmic fractions occurred in the presence of 10 μg/ml cycloheximide (Fig. 9), but the increase was less than that of controls. The extent of inhibition of RNA labeling by cycloheximide was similar using concentrations ranging from 0.4 to 50.0 μg/ml. This indicated that the alteration in RNA synthesis was a result of an effect on protein synthesis rather than a direct effect of cycloheximide on DNA transcription. Inhibition of virion labeling by cycloheximide may be in part related to this indirect inhibition of RNA synthesis during the intervals examined.

DISCUSSION

A rapid procedure for the detection of the virion RNA of RNA-containing tumor viruses is described. Short-term labeling with uridine-^{3}H minimized the contamination of crudely fractionated virions by radioactive cellular nucleic acids. Migration of the vRNA in gel slabs of polyacrylamide-agarose mixtures separated the vRNA from extraneous RNAs and allowed the comparative analysis of multiple samples.

Radioactivity was found in the RNA of completed virions within 80 min after the addition of uridine-^{3}H to the extracellular medium. Consideration of the time (less than 5 min) required for the transport, phosphorylation, and appearance of uridine-^{3}H at the site of vRNA synthesis brings the measured interval between incorporation of label and release as virion RNA to 70–75 min.

The specific interval between completion of synthesized vRNA and incorporation into virion could be less than that observed by labeling. Calculation of this interval would be best determined having a detailed knowledge of the specific activities of nucleotide precursor pools, the molecular weight (number of nucleotides) of vRNA, and the rate of elongation of the polyribonucleotide chain. Nevertheless, an estimate can be derived from the following considerations. It can be shown that total uptake of uridine-^{3}H into cells continuously exposed to label is linear for at least 120 min, and incorporation into cellular RNA likewise is linear over this interval. Essentially arithmetic accumulation of labeled vRNA was found beginning about 20 min after the first detection of labeled RNA in virions. Thus, it is unlikely that synthesis of complete strands of vRNA requires more than 20 min.

The possibly differing specific activities of the pyrimidine pools of temporarily and continuously labeled cultures did not affect the kinetics of vRNA labeling for at least 1 hour subsequent to removal of uridine-^{3}H from the culture medium. This also suggests that the radioactive vRNA observed in virions after 80 min was completed more than 1 hour before. The 70–75-min interval determined between incorporation of radioactivity and the appearance of labeled vRNA in virions must be very close to the interval between actual completion of synthesized vRNA and its extrusion in virions.

Experiments with actinomycin D are consistent with this conclusion. Actinomycin D when added immediately after a short pulse of uridine-^{3}H completely suppressed the development of labeled vRNA in virions. However, as little as 15 minutes delay in the addition of this antimetabolite allowed significant subsequent labeling of extracellular vRNA which first appears nearly an hour later. Also, if actinomycin D was added after maximal labeling rates were attained, labeling of virions continued for about 1 hour before declining. These results suggest about a 1-hour interval between the completion of vRNA and its extrusion in virions.

The noted inhibition of appearance of labeled virus by early addition of actinomycin D confirms earlier reports on the efficacy of this compound in inhibiting virus production (Temin, 1963; Bader, 1964; Duesberg and Robinson, 1967; Bases and King, 1967). Whether the synthesis of vRNA is interrupted by the direct action of actinomycin D on transcription of DNA has not been resolved. The observed inhibition by actinomycin D of the increase in radioactive cytoplasmic RNA may also influence the labeling of virion RNA. It is notable that other cytolytic RNA viruses are unaffected by actinomycin D treatment over much longer intervals than used here (Reich et al., 1961; Bader, 1964). This inhibition shortly after exposure to actinomycin D is unique -to RNA viruses of the oncogenic group.

The utter inhibition of virion RNA labeling by early addition of cycloheximide requires explanation. The slight reduction in cellular RNA synthesis by cycloheximide suggests that total inhibition of viral RNA synthesis is unlikely. However, the kinetics of inhibition of virion RNA labeling are strikingly similar to those seen after treatment with actinomycin D. Both compounds inhibit this labeling when added within 15 min after uridine-^{3}H; inhibition by either is incomplete after this time. This coincidence seems best explained by a requirement for concomitant, or nearly so, viral protein and viral RNA synthesis. A more complete explanation requires identification of the intracellular site of synthesis of the RNA of

RNA-containing tumor viruses and processes associated with this synthesis.

It is likely that sufficient virion protein accumulates to allow virus production for at least 1 hour after cessation of protein synthesis. However, Biswal *et al.* (1968) have reported accumulation of vRNA of murine sarcoma virus and MLV intracellulary within 1 hour after cycloheximide treatment. The failure of cycloheximide to prevent the entry of labeled vRNA into virions suggests that such cycloheximide-imposed accumulation of intracellular vRNA is unlikely. No such accumulation was detected in similar experiments in this laboratory using the JLSV$_5$ cells (unpublished observations). Nevertheless, the usefulness of antimetabolites in the detection of the intracellular site of synthesis of vRNA seems promising, and such studies are in progress.

ACKNOWLEDGMENTS

The author acknowledges the invaluable assistance of Nancy Brown and David Ray in the performance of the experiments described.

REFERENCES

BADER, J. P. (1964). The role of deoxyribonucleic acid in the synthesis of Rous sarcoma virus. *Virology* 22, 462–468.

BADER, J. P. (1965a). The requirement for DNA synthesis in the growth of Rous sarcoma and Rous associated viruses. *Virology* 26, 253–261.

BADER, J. P. (1965b). Transformation by Rous sarcoma virus: A requirement for DNA synthesis. *Science* 149, 757–758.

BADER, J. P. (1966a). Metabolic requirements for infection by Rous sarcoma virus. I. The transient requirement for DNA synthesis. *Virology* 29, 444–451.

BADER, J. P. (1966b). Metabolic requirements for infection by Rous sarcoma virus. II. The participation of cellular DNA. *Virology* 29, 452–461.

BADER, J. P., and STECK, T. L. (1969). An analysis of the structure of murine leukemia virus RNA. *J. Virol.* 4, 454–459.

BASES, R. E., and KING, A. S. (1967). Inhibition of Rauscher murine leukemia virus growth *in vitro* by actinomycin D. *Virology* 32, 175–183.

BISWAL, N., GRIZZARD, M. B., McCOMBS, R. M., and BENYESH-MELNICK, M. (1968). Characterization of intracellular ribonucleic acid specific for the murine sarcoma-leukemia virus complex. *J. Virol.* 2, 1346–1352.

BLAIR, C. D., and DUESBERG, P. H. (1968). Structure of Rauscher mouse leukemia virus RNA. *Nature* 220, 396–399.

DUESBERG, P. H. (1968). Physical properties of Rous sarcoma virus RNA. *Proc. Natl. Acad. Sci. U.S.* 60, 1511–1518.

DUESBERG, P. H., and BLAIR, P. B. (1966). Isolation of the nucleic acid of mouse mammary tumor virus (MTV). *Proc. Natl. Acad. Sci. U.S.* 55, 1490–1497.

DUESBERG, P. H., and CARDIFF, R. D. (1968). Structural relationships between the RNA of mammary tumor virus and those of other RNA tumor viruses. *Virology* 36, 696–700.

DUESBERG, P., and ROBINSON, W. S. (1967). Inhibition of mouse leukemia virus (MLV) replication by actinomycin D. *Virology* 31, 742–746.

ERICKSON, R. (1969). Studies on the RNA from avian myeloblastosis virus. *Virology* 37, 124–131.

HANAFUSA, H., and HANAFUSA, T. (1966). Analysis of defectiveness of Rous sarcoma virus. IV. Kinetics of RSV production. *Virology* 28, 369–378.

HAREL, J., HUPPERT, J., LACOUR, F., and HAREL, L. (1965). Demonstration of a ribonucleic acid of very high molecular weight in the avian myeloblastosis virus. *Compt. Rend. Acad. Sci. (Paris)* 261, 2266–2268.

NAKATA, Y., and BADER, J. P. (1968). Tranformation by murine sarcoma virus: Fixation (deoxyribonucleic acid synthesis) and development. *J. Virol.* 2, 1255–1261.

PEACOCK, A. C., and DINGMAN, C. W. (1967). Resolution of multiple ribonucleic acid species by polyacrylamide gel electrophoresis. *Biochemistry* 6, 1818–1827.

PEACOCK, A. C., and DINGMAN, C. W. (1968). Molecular weight estimation and separation of ribonucleic acid by electrophoresis in agarose-acrylamide composite gels. *Biochemistry* 7, 668–674.

REICH, E., FRANKLIN, R. M., SHATKIN, A. J., and TATUM, E. L. (1961). The effect of actinomycin D on cellular nucleic acid synthesis and virus production. *Science* 134, 556–557.

ROBINSON, W. S., PITKANEN, A., and RUBIN, H. (1965). The nucleic acid of the Bryan strain of Rous sarcoma virus: Purification of the virus and isolation of the nucleic acid. *Proc. Natl. Acad. Sci. U.S.* 54, 137–144.

TEMIN, N. M. (1963). The effects of actinomycin D on growth of Rous sarcoma virus *in vitro*. *Virology* 20, 577–582.

VALENTINE, A. F., and BADER, J. P. (1968). Production of virus by mammalian cells transformed by Rous sarcoma and murine sarcoma viruses. *J. Virol.* 2, 224–237.

Deoxyribonucleic Acid Polymerase of Rous Sarcoma Virus: Studies on the Mechanism of Double-Stranded Deoxyribonucleic Acid Synthesis

ANTHONY FARAS, LOIS FANSHIER, AXEL-CLAUDE GARAPIN, WARREN LEVINSON,
AND J. MICHAEL BISHOP

The virions of ribonucleic acid (RNA) tumor viruses contain at least two deoxyribonucleic acid (DNA) polymerase activities: (i) transcription of RNA into single-stranded DNA, using the RNA of the viral genome as template (1, 16), and (ii) the subsequent synthesis of double-stranded DNA (4, 5), utilizing product of the first reaction as template (6, 14). The RNA-dependent reaction results in the formation of DNA:RNA hybrids, which presumably represent intermediates in the synthesis of double-stranded DNA (7, 12, 13). However, the precise mechanism of double-stranded DNA synthesis has yet to be elucidated. The present study was undertaken to determine whether the single-stranded DNA constituent of the hybrid intermediate serves as a direct precursor of double-stranded DNA and to elucidate further the role of DNA:RNA hybrid in the enzymatic reaction.

MATERIALS AND METHODS

Reagents. ^{3}H-thymidine triphosphate (TTP), 10 to 15 Ci/mmole, was from the New England Nuclear Corp. Pancreatic ribonuclease A was from Worthington Biochemicals, Inc. Stock solutions were boiled for 10 min to inactivate any contaminating deoxyribonuclease. Pronase (B grade) was from Calbiochem. It was self-digested at 37 C for 2 hr before use. Deoxyribonucleoside triphosphates, deoxyadenosine triphosphate, deoxycytidine triphosphate, and deoxyguanosine triphosphate, were from Calbiochem. Phenol (reagent grade) was from Mal-linckrodt. Hydroxyapatite (Biol-Gel HT) was from Bio-Rad, Richmond, Calif. Nonidet P40 (NP-40) was from the Shell Chemical Co. Actinomycin D was a gift from Merck, Sharp and Dohme, Inc.

Propagation and purification of virus. The Schmidt-Ruppin strain of Rous sarcoma virus was grown in chick embryo fibroblasts and purified as described previously (2).

Extraction and purification of viral RNA. Rous sarcoma virus. RNA was extracted from purified virus with sodium dodecyl sulfate and phenol (2). The 70S RNA was isolated by zonal centrifugation through density gradients of sucrose (2, 7).

DNA polymerase reaction. Details of the enzyme reaction mixture have been reported (7). ^{3}H-TTP was used as labeled precursor. Enzymatic activity was elicited by treating virus suspensions with various concentrations of NP-40. The detergent was included in the reaction mixture, which was warmed to 37 C before addition of appropriate amounts of purified virus. Under these conditions, DNA synthesis began immediately. Determination of acid-precipitable radioactivity was accomplished as described previously (7).

Extraction and purification of enzymatic product. Reaction mixtures were treated with sodium dodecyl sulfate (0.5%, w/v) and Pronase (500 μg/ml) for 45 min at 37 C and then centrifuged through density gradients of 15 to 30% sucrose containing 0.1 M NaCl - 0.001 M ethylenediaminetetraacetic acid (EDTA)-0.02 M tris(hydroxymethyl)aminomethane (Tris)-hydrochloride, pH 7.4. Centrifugation was carried out in a Spinco SW 41 rotor at 40,000 rev/min for 180 min at 4 C. Fractions (0.3 ml) were collected, and samples were taken for determination of acid-precipitable radioactivity (7). Appropriate regions of the gradient were pooled and stored at −20 C pending further analysis.

Fractionation of DNA on hydroxyapatite. Single-stranded DNA and double-stranded DNA were separated by step-wise elution from hydroxyapatite as described previously (4). Nucleic acids were treated with ribonuclease (10 μg/ml, 3 mM EDTA, 37 C, 1 hr) to disrupt DNA:RNA hybrids. This procedure is necessitated by the fact that the elution of native hybrids from hydroxyapatite substantially overlaps that of double-stranded DNA (4). Consequently, analysis on hydroxyapatite cannot distinguish between free single-stranded DNA and that which was originally complexed to RNA.

Rate-zonal centrifugation. All analyses were carried out in density gradients of 15 to 30% sucrose containing 0.1 M NaCl-0.001 M EDTA-0.02 M Tris-hydrochloride, pH 7.4. Conditions of centrifugation are given for individual experiments.

RESULTS

Single-stranded DNA as precursor to double-stranded DNA: pulse-chase experiments with virion polymerase. The overall synthesis of DNA in vitro by Rous sarcoma virus polymerase is probably accomplished in several sequential steps (Fig. 1): (i) synthesis of a short piece of

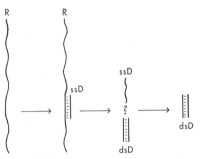

FIG. 1. *Hypothetical model for transcription of viral RNA. R, single-stranded viral RNA; ssD, single-stranded DNA; ds DNA, double-stranded DNA. This model incorporates the presently known features of the transcription of tumor virus RNA into DNA. (i) The initial reaction is RNA-dependent (1, 16), involving the synthesis of a short piece of single-stranded DNA utilizing 70S viral RNA as template and resulting in an RNA:DNA hybrid with a long tail of single-stranded RNA (7, 12); the transcribed region of viral RNA was chosen arbitrarily, and no effort has been made to portray the fact that the entire viral genome is ultimately transcribed (2a). (ii) The final reaction is probably DNA-dependent, in that it is actinomycin-sensitive (8) and capable of accepting exogenous double-stranded DNA as template (8, 9a, 13a). (iii) The final product appears to be double-stranded DNA (4, 5). (iv) Single-stranded DNA, free from viral RNA, may or may not be an intermediate in the synthesis of double-stranded DNA (9).*

single-stranded DNA, utilizing 70S viral RNA as template and resulting in a DNA:RNA hybrid with a long tail of single-stranded RNA (7); and (ii) synthesis of double-stranded DNA (4), either directly from the hybrid or by way of an intermediate form of uncertain structure (*see below*). This model gives rise to a fundamental question regarding the mechanism of double-stranded DNA synthesis: does such synthesis proceed in a conservative or a semiconservative manner, i.e., does single-stranded DNA remain in the hybrid state and function simply as template (conservative mechanism) or is it actually a direct precursor of double-stranded DNA (semiconservative mechanism)? In an effort to answer this question, we have performed "pulse-chase" experiments in which a brief period of labeling with radioactive precursor is followed by periods of "chase" with an excess of unlabeled precursor. As a matter of convenience, we have utilized an enzymatic reaction in which the rate of DNA synthesis has been reduced well below the maximum (6). This reduction was accomplished by utilizing a concentration of nucleoside triphosphate precursor (8×10^{-7} M ^{3}H-TTP) which limits the reaction rate to 1% of the maximum (6) and by treating the virus suspensions with suboptimal amounts of nonionic detergent (7). The consequence of this latter maneuver is illustrated in Fig. 2, which contrasts the kinetics of DNA synthesis elicited by 0.005 and 0.01% NP-40. At the lower concentration of detergent, detectable DNA synthesis began only after an appreciable lag (ca. 15 min) and then proceeded at a rate which was somewhat lower than that observed with the higher concentration of detergent. When analyzed by rate-zonal centrifugation and elution from hydroxyapatite, the DNA synthesized by the detergent-limited reaction (i.e., 0.005% NP-40) proved to be qualitatively similar to that synthesized at higher concentrations of detergent, although the appearance of double-stranded DNA was appreciably delayed (6; *unpublished data*).

The kinetics of representative "pulse-chase" experiments are illustrated in Fig. 3. Addition of unlabeled TTP 45 min after the onset of DNA synthesis sharply curtailed further incorporation of the radioactive precursor, although incorporation was not completely arrested until approximately 1 hr after the chase. By contrast, addition of actinomycin to the reaction mixture simultaneously with the chase resulted in the immediate cessation of incorporation. If actinomycin was present from the onset of the reaction, synthesis of DNA during the hour before the chase was reduced by a factor of two. This is a consequence

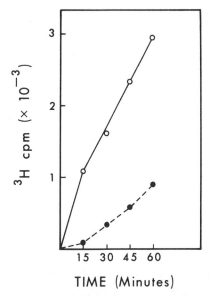

FIG. 2. *Effect of reduced detergent concentration on synthesis of DNA by Rous sarcoma virus polymerase. Standard reaction mixtures, containing 200 μg of virus protein per ml, 8 × 10⁻⁷ M ³H-thymidine triphosphate, and either 0.005% (●) or 0.01% (○) Nonidet P40 were incubated at 37 C. Samples were withdrawn at the indicated time points for determination of acid-precipitable radioactivity.*

of the previously described inhibitory effect of actinomycin on the DNA-dependent portion of the reaction (8).

Fate of single-stranded DNA during a chase. The fate of the single-stranded DNA which is labeled during the course of a pulse was followed by analysis of enzymatic product on hydroxyapatite (Fig. 4). As noted above, the detergent-limited reaction synthesized double-stranded DNA very slowly (Fig. 4, left panel). After the addition of excess unlabeled precursor (TTP), however, a major portion (ca. 75%) of the labeled DNA was converted to a double-stranded form, with a concomitant decrease in labeled single-stranded DNA (Fig. 4, right panel). Addition of actinomycin at the time of the chase completely blocked this conversion (Fig. 4, right panel). These data indicate that most of the single-stranded DNA synthesized during the initial phase of the reaction is eventually incorporated

into double-stranded DNA, presumably by serving as an unconserved template.

The conversion of single- to double-stranded DNA suggests that single-stranded DNA was continuously displaced from its initial hybrid state (Fig. 4), possibly by the ongoing synthesis of successive chains of DNA against the RNA template (*see below*; Fig. 9). It should be possible to detect this putative displacement by zonal centrifugation because the final double-stranded enzymatic product has a relatively low sedimentation velocity (7), whereas the DNA:RNA hybrid sediments rapidly (ca. 70S at early time points). A comparison by zonal centrifugation of control and "pulse-chase" reaction products is illustrated in Fig. 5 and 6. As expected, the early product (through 60 min) of the control reaction consisted primarily of the DNA:RNA hybrid which cosedimented precisely with 70S viral

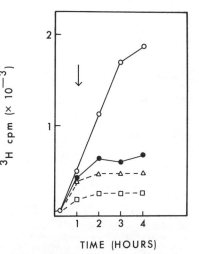

TIME (HOURS)

FIG. 3. *Pulse-chase experiments with virion polymerase. Replicate reaction mixtures were prepared with 200 μg of virus protein per ml, 8 × 10⁻⁷ M ³H-thymidine triphosphate (TTP), and 0.005% Nonidet P40. Samples were withdrawn at the indicated time points for determination of acid-precipitable radioactivity. At 60 min (arrow), three of the four reaction mixtures received additions of unlabeled TTP in 100-fold excess of the ³H-TTP. Actinomycin (50 μg/ml) was added to one of the chase reaction mixtures at the onset of the reaction and to another simultaneously with the chase of unlabeled TTP. Symbols: ○, control (not chased); ●, chase; □, chase, with actinomycin added at the onset of the reaction; △, chase, with simultaneous addition of unlabeled TTP and actinomycin at 60 min.*

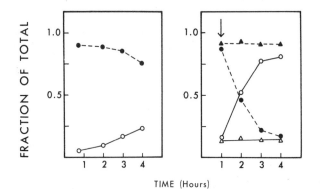

FIG. 4. *Fate of pulse-labeled DNA. Replicate reaction mixtures were prepared as for Fig. 3. Three of the four reactions were "chased" with unlabeled thymidine triphosphate at 60 min (arrow). Samples were taken at the indicated time points, extracted, and analyzed for relative content of radioactive single- and double-stranded DNA by elution from hydroxyapatite after treatment with ribonuclease (4). This procedure does not distinguish single-stranded DNA contained in hybrid structures from that which is not complexed with RNA (4). The left-hand panel illustrates the results of a control (not "chased") reaction. Symbols:* ●, *single-stranded DNA;* ○, *double-stranded DNA. The right-hand panel illustrates the results of the chased reactions. Symbols:* ●, *single-stranded DNA in chased reaction;* ○, *double-stranded DNA in chased reaction;* ▲, *single-stranded DNA in chased reaction containing actinomycin (50 μg/ml, added at the time of the chase);* △, *double-stranded DNA in the chased reaction containing actinomycin.*

RNA (Fig. 5a). By 2 hr, there was a slight but consistent discrepancy between the sedimentation velocity of 70S viral RNA and that of the hybrid enzymatic product (Fig. 5d). This discrepancy was even more apparent at 4 hr (Fig. 5e), although the bulk of the hybrid population was still coincident with the 70S viral RNA in the sucrose gradient.

These progressive changes in sedimentation velocity were accentuated by a chase (Fig. 6). At 4 hr, none of the labeled enzymatic product cosedimented with 70S viral RNA (Fig. 6e). Nevertheless, an appreciable portion of the product (ca. 40 to 50%) still sedimented more rapidly than the slowly sedimenting population which contains the final double-stranded product of the reaction (4).

Ribonuclease treatment of the rapidly sedimenting DNA isolated from control and pulse-chase reactions converted these DNA species to a low-molecular-weight form (Fig. 7). Thus, all of the rapidly sedimenting DNA present at 4 hr in both the control and the "pulse-chase" reactions consisted of low-molecular-weight DNA associated with high-molecular-weight single-stranded RNA. These observations do not conform to the expectation that the conversion of single- to double-stranded DNA is accompanied by displacement of the former from

the DNA:RNA hybrid and prompted us to examine the secondary structure of the DNA in question by analysis on hydroxyapatite. In agreement with our previously published results (4), the rapidly sedimenting hybrid isolated from either a control or a pulse-chase reaction at an early time point contained only single-stranded DNA (Fig. 8c). At 4 hr, however, the hybrid from a control reaction contained an appreciable amount (ca. 25%) of double-stranded DNA (Fig. 8e), and the hybrid from a "pulse-chase" reaction contained primarily double-stranded DNA (ca. 70%; Fig. 8g). In both cases, treatment of the hybrid with alkali completely denatured the double-stranded DNA constituent (Fig. 8f and h). These observations indicate that conversion of single- to double-stranded DNA occurred in association with the initial template for DNA synthesis, the 70S viral RNA, and account in large measure for the fact that a chase did not completely displace radiolabel from the rapidly sedimenting form of enzymatic product.

Actinomycin, which completely inhibits the DNA-dependent portions of virion-associated DNA synthesis (8), blocked the conversion of pulse-labeled single-stranded DNA into double-stranded DNA (Fig. 4). Consequently, hybrid synthesized in the presence of actinomycin con-

46

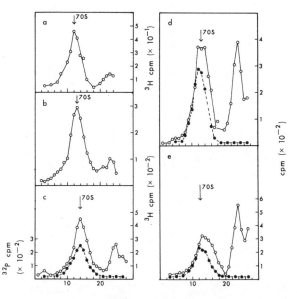

FRACTION NUMBER

Fig. 5. *Rate-zonal centrifugation of enzymatic product from a control reaction. A standard reaction mixture was prepared with 300 μg of virus protein and* 4×10^{-6}M *^{3}H-thymidine triphosphate (TTP). This concentration of ^{3}H-TTP was required to obtain sufficient enzymatic product to allow multiple centrifugal analyses. Samples were withdrawn at the indicated time points, extracted with sodium dodecyl sulfate and Pronase, and analyzed by centrifugation through density gradients of sucrose in an SW 41 rotor. ^{32}P-labeled 70S viral RNA was included as a sedimentation reference. (a) At 15 min. The 70S sedimentation marker is not illustrated but was coincident with the rapidly sedimenting enzymatic product. (b) At 30 min. The 70S sedimentation on marker is not illustrated but was coincident with the rapidly sedimenting enzymatic product. (c) At 60 min. (d) At 120 min. (e) At 240 min. Symbols: ○, ^{3}H-labeled enzymatic product; ●, ^{32}P-labeled 70S viral RNA.*

tained only single-stranded DNA at all time points during the course of both control and pulse-chase reactions (Table 1).

DISCUSSION

Hypothetical model for DNA synthesis. On the basis of the preceding data, we propose a preliminary model for the synthesis of DNA by the virion polymerases (Fig. 9). This model incorporates the four principle features of the reaction which have been elucidated to date. (i) The initial event is synthesis of short segments of single-stranded DNA, utilizing 70S RNA as template and resulting in the formation of a DNA:RNA hybrid. (ii) A portion of the DNA contained in this hybrid is accessible to digestion by the single strand-specific endonuclease of *Neurospora* (9), i.e., the hybrid apparently possesses branches of single-stranded DNA. (iii) Single-stranded DNA serves as template and precursor for the synthesis of double-stranded DNA. (iv) The synthesis of double-stranded DNA appears to occur, or at least to be initiated, in association with the viral RNA (Fig. 8 and reference 8).

We suggest that the branched hybrid results from displacement of a completed (or partially completed) DNA strand by the growth of a newly initiated strand. In this regard, the model is similar to that proposed by Manly et al. (9) and draws upon familiar mechanisms for the synthesis of single-stranded viral RNA (15).

To accomodate our observation that the synthesis of double-stranded DNA occurs in association with the DNA:RNA hybrid (Fig.

47

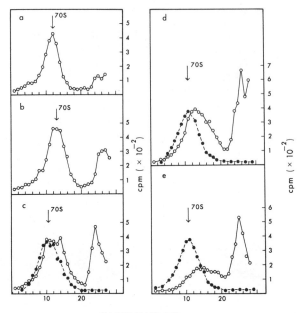

FIG. 6. *Rate-zonal centrifugation of enzymatic product from a chased reaction. A reaction mixture identical to that described for Fig. 5 was prepared. After 15 min of incubation at 37 C, unlabeled thymidine triphosphate (TTP) was added in 100-fold excess of the ³H-TTP. Samples of the reaction mixture were extracted and analyzed by rate-zonal centrifugation as in Fig. 5. ³²P-labeled 70S viral RNA was included as a sedimentation reference. (a) At 15 min. Sample taken immediately before the chase. (b) At 30 min. (c) At 60 min. (d) At 120 min. (e) At 240 min. Symbols: ○, ³H-labeled enzymatic product; ●, ³²P-labeled 70S viral RNA.*

6 and 8), we propose that DNA synthesis is initiated against the partially displaced single strands before they are released from the hybrid. We assume that, as in other instances (3), the synthesis of DNA is unidirectional (i.e., from the 5′ terminus towards the 3′ terminus). Consequently, a partially displaced strand can serve as template for further DNA synthesis only if there are repeated initiations in the manner suggested by Okazaki et al. for the replication of bacterial DNA (10). These initiations, in turn, would give rise to covalent gaps in the nascent DNA strand which would have to be closed by the action of a ligase enzyme (11). According to the model, double-stranded DNA could not be completed until after its release from the hybrid. Moreover, disruption of the hybrid by hydrolysis with ribonuclease in low concentrations of electrolytes would release incomplete

(i.e., partially single-stranded) double-stranded DNA (Fig. 9). Attempts to identify and isolate DNA of this sort from disrupted hybrid are now in progress.

The foregoing proposals are clearly provisional and are subject to the criticism that the data were obtained with crude enzyme preparations. Such preparations may be contaminated with endonucleases and other possible sources of artifact. However, we have shown that, under the conditions used for these experiments, the Rous sarcoma virus virion is not disrupted, the viral genome (i.e., the primary template for DNA synthesis) remains intact, and no deoxyribonuclease active against double-stranded DNA is detectable in the reaction mixture (*in preparation*). Consequently, DNA synthesis is effected by an ostensibly undisturbed and coordinated series of enzymatic reactions which may well

48

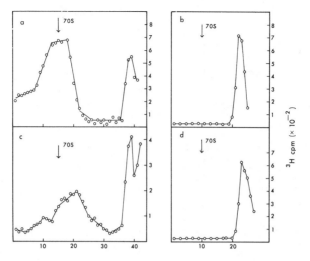

FRACTION NUMBER

FIG. 7. *Effect of ribonuclease on rapidly sedimenting enzymatic product. Reaction mixtures similar to those described for Fig. 5 and 6 were prepared in duplicate. One reaction was chased with unlabeled TTP at 15 min. After 240 min of incubation, the entire reaction mixtures were extracted and centrifuged through sucrose density gradients. The rapidly sedimenting material was isolated from the gradients, treated with ribonuclease (10 µg/ml, 3 mm ethylenediamine tetraacetic acid), and analyzed by recentrifugation under the same conditions as before.* ^{32}P-labeled 70S viral RNA was added directly to the samples before the initial centrifugation, but was centrifuged in a separate bucket for the second analysis to avoid degradation by the ribonuclease. (a) Control reaction. (b) Control reaction; 70S hybrid isolated from the gradient illustrated in (a), treated with ribonuclease, and recentrifuged. (c) Chase reaction. (d) Chase reaction; 70S hybrid isolated from the gradient illustrated in (c), treated with ribonuclease, and recentrifuged.

approximate the circumstances that follow viral infection. The issue can only be resolved by comparisons between the present experimental system and purified, template-dependent enzymes (*in preparation*).

Sedimentation properties of the DNA:RNA hybrid. The initial product of enzymatic synthesis is a DNA:RNA hybrid which is composed of a small fragment of nascent DNA hydrogen-bonded to 70S viral RNA. The sedimentation velocity of this material is apparently determined solely by the RNA constituent (7). Consequently, the hybrid co-sediments with 70S viral RNA (Fig. 5). As the enzymatic reaction progresses, however, there is a detectable reduction in the sedimentation velocity of at least a portion of the hybrid population (Fig. 5d and e). Moreover, the hybrid which retains label after a prolonged chase has a considerably reduced sedimentation velocity (Fig. 6e). Much of the labeled DNA contained in the latter form of

hybrid elutes from hydroxyapatite as if it were double-stranded (Fig. 8g), and we have suggested that this DNA represents branches of partially completed double-strands which are still associated with the hybrid intermediate (Fig. 9). It seems reasonable to expect that the addition of a double-stranded branch to the DNA: RNA hybrid in this manner would retard its sedimentation through sucrose and that the extent of this retardation would be determined by the length and number of double-stranded branches. After a chase period, any label still remaining associated with hybrid structures would be in the double-stranded branches nearest to completion, and this portion of the hybrid population would be most retarded in its sedimentation velocity (Fig. 6e).

Kinetics of DNA synthesis at 0.005% NP-40. RNA tumor viruses must be treated with a non-ionic detergent to elicit DNA polymerase activity. The only possible exception to this is the

49

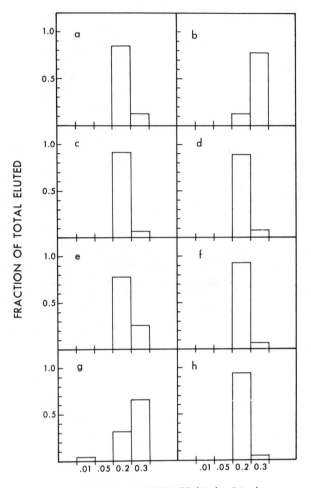

FIG. 8. *Analysis of rapidly sedimenting enzymatic product on hydroxyapatite. Control and chase reactions were performed as described for Fig. 5 and 6. Samples were withdrawn at 15 and 240 min for extraction and centrifugation through sucrose gradients. The results were essentially as illustrated in Fig. 5 and 6. Rapidly sedimenting product was isolated from the gradients, treated with ribonuclease (10 μg/ml, 3 mM ethylenediaminetetraacetic acid, 1 hr, 37 C) to release the DNA from RNA, and analyzed by elution from hydroxyapatite (4). Single-stranded DNA of fd phage and double-stranded avian DNA were included in the analyses as controls (4). (a) Single-stranded fd DNA. (b) Double-stranded DNA from chick fibroblasts. (c) At 15 min, rapidly sedimenting product from either control or chase reaction. The results were identical. (d) Same samples as c but treated with NaOH (0.6 N, 1 hr, 37 C). (e) At 240 min, rapidly sedimenting product from control reaction. (f) Same sample as e but treated with NaOH. (g) At 240 min, rapidly sedimenting product from chase reaction. (h) Same sample as g but treated with NaOH.*

case of virus which has been stored for an appreciable period of time (1). This requirement for detergent probably involves partial or complete disruption of the viral envelope, presumably to allow penetration of the nucleoside triphosphates to the interior of the virion. Consequently,

TABLE 1. *Nature of the DNA in rapidly sedimenting hybrid*

Determination	Single-stranded DNA (%)	Double-stranded DNA (%)
Control[a]...	86	14
Chase[b]...............	34	66
Chase plus actinomycin[c]........	83	17

[a] Rapidly sedimenting hybrid was isolated at 4 hr from a control reaction and analyzed on hydroxyapatite as described for Fig. 8.

[b] Reaction was chased at 15 min with unlabeled thymidine triphosphate (see Fig. 6). Rapidly sedimenting hybrid was isolated and analyzed as in footnote a.

[c] Reaction was carried out in the presence of actinomycin D (50 μg/ml) and chased at 15 min. Rapidly sedimenting hybrid was isolated and analyzed as in footnote a.

extremely low concentrations of detergent elicit only limited amounts of enzymatic activity (7) and may also appreciably delay the onset of detectable DNA synthesis (Fig. 2). Whether this represents limitation of precursor access to the enzyme or some other structural constraint on enzymatic activity, or both, is presently indeterminate.

Characteristics of the chase reaction. Addition of large excesses of unlabeled TTP do not immediately arrest the incorporation of ^{3}H-TTP into an acid-precipitable state unless DNA-dependent synthesis is inhibited with a high concentration of actinomycin (Fig. 3). This observation suggests that the RNA-dependent reaction responds to a chase more quickly than does the DNA-dependent reaction, but no explanation for such differential response is apparent at present.

The transition of radioactive DNA from a single- to double-stranded form after a chase is never complete (Fig. 4). We cannot presently explain this observation. It could represent an artifact of the in vitro reaction or a biochemically significant restriction on the extent to which the single-stranded product is copied by viral DNA-dependent polymerase.

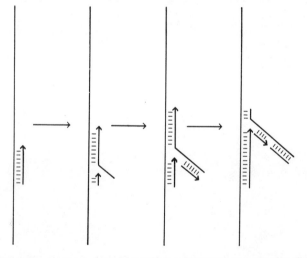

FIG. 9. *Hypothetical model for the synthesis of double-stranded DNA by virion polymerase. Horizontal bars represent hydrogen bonds. The growing termini of nascent DNA chains are indicated by arrowheads. The long bar represents single-stranded RNA template, the transcribed region of which was chosen arbitrarily. DNA synthesis was assumed to be unidirectional.*

ACKNOWLEDGMENTS

We are indebted to Jean Jackson, Barbara Evans, Joyce Skiles, and Nancy Quintrell for assistance, to K. Manly and D. Baltimore for communication of data before publication, and to L. Levintow for support and editorial assistance.

This work was supported by Public Health Service grants AI 08864 and AI 06862 from the National Institute of Allergy and Infectious Diseases and by grants from the California Division of the American Cancer Society (no. 483) and the Cancer Research Coordinating Committee of the University of California.

LITERATURE CITED

1. Baltimore, D. 1970. RNA-dependent DNA polymerase in virions of RNA tumour viruses. Nature (London) 226:1209–1211.

2. Bishop, J. M., W. E. Levinson, N. Quintrell, D. Sullivan, L. Fanshier, and J. Jackson. 1970. The low molecular weight RNA's of Rous sarcoma virus. I. The 4S RNA. Virology 42:182–195.

2a. Duesberg, P. H., and E. Canaani. 1970. Complementarity between Rous sarcoma virus (RSV) RNA and the in vitro synthetized DNA of the virus-associated DNA polymerase. Virology 42:783–788.

3. Englund, P. T., M. P. Deutscher, T. M. Jovin, R. B. Kelly, W. R. Cozzarelli, and A. Kornberg. 1968. Cold Spring Harbor Symp. Quant. Biol. 33:1–9.

4. Fanshier, L., A.-C. Garapin, J. McDonnell, A. Faras, W. Levinson, and J. M. Bishop. 1971. Deoxyribonucleic acid polymerase associated with avian tumor viruses: secondary structure of the deoxyribonucleic acid product. J. Virol. 7:77–86.

5. Fujinaga, K., J. T. Parsons, J. W. Beard, D. Beard, and M. Green. 1970. Mechanism of carcinogenesis by RNA tumor viruses. III. Formation of RNA : DNA complex and duplex DNA molecules by the DNA polymerase(s) of avian myeloblastosis virus. Proc. Nat. Acad. Sci. U.S.A. 67:1432–1439.

6. Garapin, A.-C., L. Fanshier, J. Leong, J. Jackson, W. Levinson, and J. M. Bishop. 1970. Deoxyribonucleic acid polymerases of Rous sarcoma virus: kinetics of deoxyribonucleic acid synthesis and specificity of the products. J. Virol. 7:227–232.

7. Garapin, A.-C., J. P. McDonnell, W. Levinson, N. Quintrell, L. Fanshier, and J. M. Bishop. 1970. Deoxyribonucleic acid

polymerase associated with Rous sarcoma virus and avian myeloblastosis virus: properties of the enzyme and its product. J. Virol. 6:589–598.

8. McDonnell, J. P., A.-C. Garapin, W. E. Levinson, N. Quintrell, L. Fanshier, and J. M. Bishop. 1970. DNA polymerase associated with Rous sarcoma virus: delineation of two reactions with actinomycin. Nature (London) 228:433–435.

9. Manly, K. F., D. F. Smoler, E. Bromfield, and D. Baltimore. 1971. Forms of deoxyribonucleic acid produced by virions of the ribonucleic acid tumor viruses. J. Virol. 7:106–111.

9a. Mizutani, S., D. Boettiger, and H. M. Temin. 1970. A DNA-dependent DNA polymerase and a DNA endonuclease in virions of Rous sarcoma virus. Nature (London) 228:424–427.

10. Okazaki, R., T. Okazaki, K. Sakabe, K. Sugimoto, R. Kainuma, A. Gugino, and N. Iwatsuki. 1968. In vivo mechanism of DNA chain growth. Cold Spring Harbor Symp. Quant. Biol. 33:129–143.

11. Richardson, C. C. 1969. Enzymes in DNA metabolism. Annu. Rev. Biochem. 38:795–840.

12. Rokutanda, M., H. Rokutanda, M. Green, K. Fujinaga, R. K. Ray, and C. Gurgo. 1970. Formation of viral RNA: DNA hybrid molecules by the DNA polymerase of sarcomaleukemia viruses. Nature (London) 227:1026–1028.

13. Spiegelman, S., A. Burny, M. R. Das, J. Keydar, J. Schlom, M. Travnicek, and K. Watson. 1970. Characterization of the products of RNA-directed DNA polymerases in oncogenic RNA viruses. Nature (London) 227:563–567.

13a. Spiegelman, S., A. Burny, M. R. Das, J. Keydar, J. Schlom, M. Travnicek, and K. Watson. 1970. DNA-directed DNA polymerase activity in oncogenic RNA viruses. Nature (London) 227:1039–1031.

14. Spiegelman, S., A. Burny, M. R. Das, J. Keydar, J. Schlom, M. Travnicek, and K. Watson. 1970. Synthetic DNA-RNA hybrids and RNA-DNA duplexes as templates for the polymerases of the oncogenic RNA viruses. Nature (London) 228:430–432.

15. Stavis, R. L., and J. T. August. 1970. The biochemistry of RNA bacteriophage replication. Annu. Rev. Biochem. 39:527–560.

16. Temin, H. M., and S. Mizutani. 1970. RNA-dependent DNA polymerase in virions of Rous sarcoma virus. Nature (London) 226:1211–1213.

Properties of a Soluble DNA Polymerase Isolated from Rous Sarcoma Virus

PETER DUESBERG, KLAUS V. D. HELM, AND ELI CANAANI

The DNA polymerase associated with avian and murine RNA tumor viruses (1, 2) accepts different kinds of nucleic acids as templates. The enzyme was originally found to be RNA-dependent with endogenous viral RNA as template (1-3). Later, it was found that both native and denatured double-stranded DNAs from various sources (4-8), as well as synthetic nucleic acids (4, 9), could serve as templates. It was therefore of interest whether the enzyme exhibits template specificity for natural RNAs, i.e., whether it prefers tumor virus RNA over RNAs from other sources; whether the DNA polymerase activities primed by endogenous viral RNA, by natural DNAs, or by synthetic nucleic acids are common to a single enzyme, to modifications of one enzyme, or to different enzymes was also of interest. It had also not been determined whether the viral DNA polymerase corresponds to any of the known structural proteins of the virus. Such questions may be answered by means of a soluble and purified viral DNA polymerase. This report describes the isolation and some properties of a soluble DNA polymerase from two strains of Rous Sarcoma Virus (RSV).

Abbreviations: RSV, Rous sarcoma virus; RSV-A and RSV-C, the serological subgroups A and C of RSV, respectively; PR RSV, Prague strain; SR RSV, Schmidt-Ruppin strain; DTT, dithiothreitol; BSA, bovine serum albumin.

MATERIALS AND METHODS

Solutions

Standard buffer contains 0.1 M NaCl–0.01 M Tris (pH 7.4)–1 mM EDTA; low-salt buffer for DEAE-cellulose chromatography is 0.05 M Tris (pH 7.4)–0.01 M MgCl$_2$–0.02 M KCl–0.2 mM EDTA–1 mM dithiothreitol (DTT)–5% glycerol; disruption buffer is 0.01 M Tris (pH 8.0)–2 mM EDTA–1 mM DTT–0.02 M KCl (for DEAE-cellulose chromatography) or 0.1 M KCl (for sedimentation).

Viruses

Growth, radioactive labeling, and purification of PR RSV-C and SR RSV-A followed published procedures (10–12). Medium for amino acid labeling (10) was modified to contain 1% calf serum, 1% chick serum, 1% dimethyl sulfoxide, and the glutamine concentration of normal medium 199. After appropriate dilution with standard buffer, purified virus was layered over a 2-cm column of 30% glycerol containing 0.01 M Tris (pH 8.0)–1 mM EDTA–1.5 mM 2-mercaptoethanol and centrifuged in a Spinco SW50.1 rotor for 30 min at 46,000 rpm (at 5°C) onto a cushion of 85% glycerol containing the same buffer. The virus, collected at the interface, was stored at −20°C. Virus concentration was determined by measuring the A_{260} in standard buffer containing 0.2% sodium dodecyl sulfate; the (SDS) A_{260}/A_{280} ratio was 1.15–1.2.

DNA polymerase assay

Standard assays were done in 50 μl, as previously described (3), but the concentration of [^{3}H]dTTP was 1.25 × 10^{-6} M (10 Ci/mmol, New England Nuclear) and 5 μg of denatured (24 hr, 0.2 N KOH, 20°C) salmon DNA in 0.01 M Tris (pH 8.0)–1 mM EDTA was included. The final concentrations of KCl and Triton X-100 varied slightly depending on the experiment. Incubation was for 1–2 hr at 38°C. [^{3}H]dTTP incorporated into DNA was precipitated by the addition of 100 μg of yeast RNA and 10 volumes of 5% trichloroacetic acid (TCA). After 10 min at 0°C, the precipitate was poured onto Millipore filters that had been soaked in a saturated solution of pyrophosphate, and washed 4 times with 5% TCA. Radioactivity was counted in a toluene-based scintillation fluid, and background (80 ± 10 cpm/filter) was subtracted.

RESULTS

Solubilization of the virus-associated DNA polymerase

To solubilize the DNA polymerase of either strain, a virus solution in (about) 50% buffered glycerol was incubated for 15 min at 38°C with 3–5 volumes of disruption buffer containing Triton X-100 at a final concentration of 0.5%. After centrifugation (< 1 ml) in a polycarbonate tube at 150,000 × g for 15 min, the supernatant contained 75% ± 4% (average of 5 preparations ± SE) of the enzymatic activity of an uncentrifuged solution. Similar experiments with radioactive virus, which contained amino acid-labeled protein (10) or glucosamine-labeled glycoprotein (11), indicated that about 80% ± 5% (average of 4 preparations ± SE) of the viral protein and the glycoprotein remained in the supernatant. Since under the same conditions of centrifugation untreated virus was pelleted, the enzymatic activity and viral proteins in the supernatant must have been released from intact virus in a soluble form.

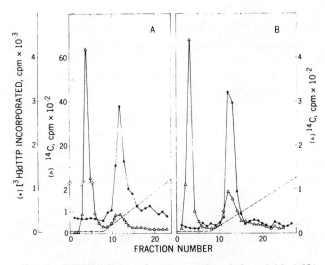

Fig. 1. DEAE-cellulose chromatography of the soluble DNA polymerase derived from [¹⁴C]amino acid-labeled (A) or [¹⁴C]-glucosamine-labeled (B) PR RSV-C. (A) 30 μl of PR RSV-C (18 A_{260}/ml) and 20 μl of [¹⁴C]amino acid-labeled PR RSV-C (about 100,000 cpm), 0.5 ml of disruption buffer containing 0.02 M KCl, and 25 μl of Triton X-100 (10% v/v) were processed and centrifuged (150,000 × g) as described for Fig. 2A. The supernatant was applied (at 5°C) to a DEAE-cellulose column (3 × 0.6 cm) equilibrated in buffer. After the column was washed with several ml of buffer, a linear KCl gradient in the same buffer was applied and 10-min (about 1-ml) fractions were collected. Analysis of the fractions was as described for Fig. 2A. (B) Same as for A, but 20 μl of [¹⁴C]glucosamine-labeled PR RSV-C (about 100,000 cpm) was used. The extremes of the KCl gradient (- - -) represent 0.02 M KCl and 0.6 M KCl.

Chromatography of the soluble DNA polymerase on DEAE-cellulose

DEAE-cellulose chromatography of the soluble DNA polymerase of [^{14}C]amino acid-labeled virus, corresponding to about 200 μg of viral protein, is shown in Fig. 1A. About 30% of the starting enzymatic activity eluted with about 2% (4 μg) of the viral protein at 0.15–0.2 M KCl. Some enzymatic activity eluted at higher KCl concentrations. Since 70% of the starting enzymatic activity was lost, this corresponds to a 15-fold enrichment of the enzyme. Because 80% of the [^{14}C]protein applied to the column was recovered, it may be concluded that the enzyme represents, at most, 2% of the soluble [^{14}C]-proteins of the virus. Fig. 1B illustrates that about 30% of the radioactive glycoprotein (11) of solubilized virus that eluted from the column cochromatographed with the viral DNA polymerase. Elution from DEAE-cellulose at 0.15–0.2 M KCl indicates that the enzyme has an isoelectric point below 6 (13), which is similar to that of other nucleic acid polymerases (14) of similar size (see below).

Sedimentation coefficient of the solubilized viral DNA polymerase before and after incubation with RNase

The DNA polymerase sedimented as a single component, with an estimated (15) $s_{20,w}$ of 8 S based on the 4.3 S value of a bovine serum albumin ([^{14}C]BSA) (16) marker (see Fig. 4A). After incubation with pancreatic RNase, the $s_{20,w}$ of the enzyme was reduced to 6 S (see Fig. 4B). The recovery of DNA polymerase activity after sucrose gradient sedimentation was 80% ± 5% (average of 4 experiments ±SE) without RNase treatment and from 40 to 80% after RNase treatment. The enzyme had a half-life in the gradient solution of $\geq$ 4 weeks at 5°C.

The molecular weight of the 8S DNA polymerase can be estimated by the formula $s_{w_1}/s_{w_2} := (MW_1/MW_2)^{2/3}$ (17) to be about 170,000 (BSA standard = 67,000) (16), and that of the 6S DNA polymerase to be about 110,000. The difference between the estimated weights of the 8S and the 6S forms of the DNA polymerase may be due to the removal by RNase of small pieces of enzyme-associated RNA.

Hydrodynamic and pherographic analyses of the 8S and the 6S viral DNA polymerase and other soluble components of the virus

It is shown in Fig. 2A that the 8S DNA polymerase did not correspond to a distinct peak of soluble [^{14}C]protein of the virus. The enzymatic activity overlapped with a [^{14}C]protein component that had a slightly higher $s_{20,w}$ than the enzymatic activity and consisted of about 12% of the radioactive protein in the gradient. This component was identified (11) as an "8S" glycoprotein complex; it will be referred to here as 9S

56

component (Fig. 2B, C) based on a 4.3S BSA standard. (The previous estimate (11) was based on tRNA, assumed to be 4S.) About 85% of the [^{14}C]protein sedimented more slowly than the 8S DNA polymerase, at about 1–2 S (Fig. 2A, C). Both the $s_{20,w}$ (11) and the electrophoretic properties (not shown, ref. 10) of this material indicated that it was the viral group-specific antigen. The three peak fractions (80%) of the 8S DNA polymerase in Fig. 2A cosedimented with about 5% of the soluble [^{14}C]protein, representing a 15-fold purification of the enzyme.

If the $s_{20,w}$ of the DNA polymerase was reduced to 6 S by treatment with RNase (Fig. 2C), the sedimentation distribution of the major viral protein components was not significantly altered; however, the three peak fractions (80%) of the enzymatic activity cosedimented with only 2% of the viral [^{14}C]proteins (Fig. 2C). This represents a 40-fold purification of the enzyme. Fig. 3A shows electrophoresis of the [^{14}C]protein that cosedimented with the 6S DNA polymerase shown in Fig. 2C. Unfractionated [^{3}H]amino acid-labeled virus was added to provide electrophoretic markers for the major structural proteins of the virus, which included the proteins of the group-specific antigen gs$_1$, gs$_2$, and gs$_3$, and the two viral glycoproteins, I (37,000 daltons) and II (105,000 daltons) (11). The majority of the [^{14}C]protein had the same electrophoretic mobility as the glycoproteins, II and I (see Fig. 3B) (11); very little ^{14}C coelectrophoresed with the components of the group-specific antigen. In addition, at least one new ^{14}C peak appeared in the gel, labeled X (Fig. 3A); it had not been identified previously (10, 11). A very similar electrophoretic pattern was obtained when the [^{14}C]protein that cochromatographed with the enzyme on DEAE-cellulose was analyzed under these conditions (not shown). It can be deduced from these experiments that the DNA polymerase is not identical with the group-specific antigen of the virus.

Cosedimentation of the 8S DNA polymerase and the soluble [^{14}C]glycoprotein of the virus is shown in Fig. 2B. The 8S polymerase overlapped with 25% of the 9S glycoprotein complex, whereas the 6S DNA polymerase overlapped with only 10% of the soluble [^{14}C]glycoprotein (Fig. 2D). Sedimentation of the enzymatic activity after overnight precipitation in 60% ammonium sulfate in the presence of 50 μg of BSA did not change the relative sedimentation distributions of the enzyme and the glycoprotein (not shown).

Electrophoresis of the [^{14}C]glycoprotein that cosedimented with the 6S DNA polymerase is shown in Fig. 3B. More than 90% of this [^{14}C]glycoprotein coelectrophoresed with the known glycoproteins I and II of unfractionated virus (11); no new distinct glycoprotein component appeared. The same electrophoretic pattern was obtained when the peak fractions

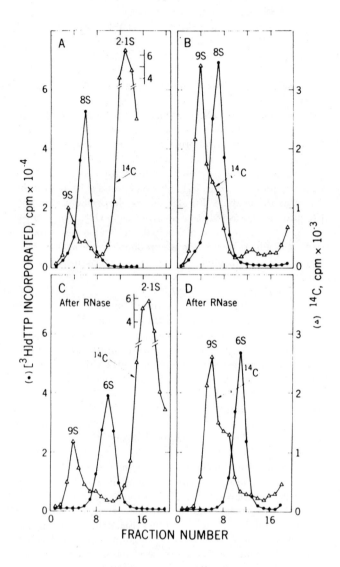

Fɪɢ. 2. Sucrose gradient sedimentation of the soluble DNA polymerase of PR RSV-C before (A, B) and after (C, D) RNase treatment. (A) 750,000 cpm of [^{14}C]amino acid-labeled PR RSV-C, 30 μl of PR RSV-C in 50% buffered glycerol at a concentration of 18 A_{260}/ml, 200 μl of disruption buffer, and 15 μl of Triton X-100 (10% v/v) were incubated at 38°C for 15 min, then centrifuged in a Spinco 40 rotor at 40,000 rpm (20°C) for 15 min in a polycarbonate tube. The supernatant was layered on a linear sucrose gradient (15–30%) containing 0.1 M KCl–0.01 M Tris-(pH 8.0)–1 mM EDTA 0.2 mM DTT–0.2% Triton X-100. The gradient was poured over a 0.3- to 0.4-ml cushion of 65% sucrose in the same buffer. Centrifugation was in a polyallomer tube in a Spinco SW65 rotor at 20°C for 9 hr at 65,000 rpm. 12-drop fractions were collected. 10-μl aliquots were assayed for polymerase activity during a 90-min incubation period. ^{14}C was determined by placing appropriate aliquots in toluene-based scintillation fluid containing 20% NCS (Nuclear-Chicago), and counting in a Tri-Carb scintillation counter. (B) [^{14}C]-glucosamine-labeled PR RSV-C containing about 250,000 cpm was mixed with 30 μl of PR RSV-C (18 A_{260}/ml) and processed as described for A. (C) Same as A, but 1 μg of pancreatic RNase (heated at 100°C for 5 min) was included in the disruption mixture. (D) Same as B, but disrupted in the presence of pancreatic RNase as described for C and centrifugation was only for 7 hr.

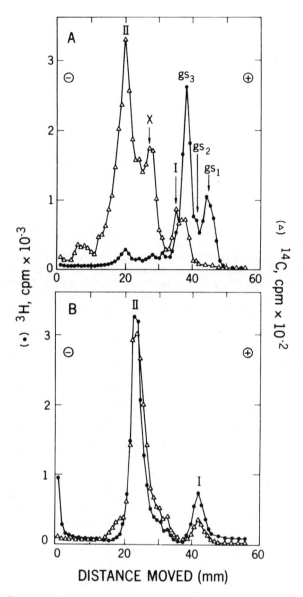

Fig. 3. Electrophoretic analysis of the [¹⁴C]amino acid- or [¹⁴C]glucosamine-labeled material of solubilized virus that co-sediments with the viral DNA polymerase. (*A*) Aliquots of fractions 9–11 (Fig. 2*C*) of [¹⁴C]amino acid-labeled virus were precipitated with 5 vol of ethanol and 50 μg of BSA. The precipitate was mixed with an appropriate amount of unfractionated [³H]-amino acid-labeled virus to provide electrophoretic markers and analyzed by electrophoresis in 5% sodium dodecyl sulfate-polyacrylamide gels as described (11). (*B*) Aliquots of fractions 10–12 (Fig. 2*D*) were precipitated as described for *A*. Prior to electrophoresis, unfractionated [³H]glucosamine-labeled PR RSV-C was added to provide glycoprotein reference markers (11).

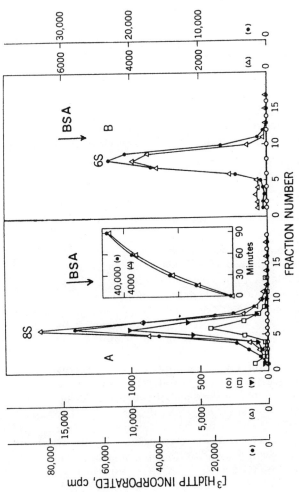

FIG. 4. Analysis of the template activities of various nucleic acids for the 8S (A) and the 6S (B) viral DNA polymerase activity. Sucrose gradient sedimentation of the soluble DNA polymerase was as described for Fig. 2A, B. The [¹⁴C]BSA, noted by an *arrow*, was present as a marker. (A) 10-μl aliquots of each fraction were incubated for 90 min with either 5 μg of salmon DNA (●—●) or 2.5 μg of 60–70S PR RSV-C RNA, (△—△), or 2.5 μg of heat-dissociated (12, 18) 60–70S PR RSV RNA (▼—▼), or 2 μg of tobacco mosaic virus RNA (□—□), or no added nucleic acid (○—○) in the standard DNA polymerase assay. Three μg of influenza virus RNA had essentially the same template activity as 2.5 μg of heat-dissociated RSV RNA (not shown). Preparation of 60–70S PR RSV RNA: PR RSV-C RNA (12, 18) was incubated in 250 μl of 0.01 M Tris (pH 7.4)–0.15 M NaCl–2 mM MgCl₂ that contained 10 μg of DNase (RNase-free) for 15 min at 38°C and 1 hr at room temperature to degrade associated DNA (22). It was then diluted with 1 ml of standard buffer containing 0.2% sodium dodecyl sulfate, extracted once with phenol, and, after ethanol precipitation, the 60–70S PR RSV-C RNA was prepared by sucrose gradient sedimentation (12). The insert shows the rate of [³H]dTTP incorporation by 10-μl aliquots of fraction 6 in the presence of 60–70S PR RSV RNA or salmon DNA. (B) RNase treatment was as described for Fig. 2. The respective fractions were tested as described for A.

61

of the 9S [^{14}C]glycoprotein component that did not sediment with enzymatic activity were analyzed (not shown), or when the [^{14}C]glycoprotein that cochromatographed with the enzyme on DEAE-cellulose (Fig. 2A) was electrophoresed (not shown). Results very similar to those described for PR RSV-C were obtained with SR RSV-A.

It may be concluded that the 6S DNA polymerase differs from 90% of the viral glycoprotein. The 10% of the viral glycoprotein that could not be separated from the 6S DNA polymerase by our methods had the same electrophoretic distribution as the two known glycoproteins of the virus.

Template specificity of the soluble DNA polymerase

The soluble DNA polymerase presented an opportunity to examine whether the enzyme was able to use added RNA templates, and whether it preferred 60–70S PR RSV RNA over other RNAs. This question could not be answered previously because the enzyme had not been solubilized, nor was it experimentally possible to eliminate the endogenous RNA template without at the same time affecting added natural RNA templates.

The 60–70S RNA of PR RSV-C was found in different experiments to have, per unit weight (saturation curves were not determined), 10–40% of the template activity of salmon DNA for both the 8S and the 6S DNA polymerase (Fig. 4A, B). The rate with the peak fraction of enzyme for native RSV RNA- and salmon DNA-primed enzymatic activities of the 8S DNA polymerase were indistinguishable (Fig. 4A). Heat-dissociated 60–70S PR RSV RNA (12, 18) had only 2–6% (range of four experiments) of the template activity of native 60–70S RNA (Fig. 4A). Other natural RNAs like tobacco mosaic virus RNA had 2%, and influenza virus RNA 5%, of the template activity of 60–70S PR RSV RNA for the 8S DNA polymerase (Fig. 4A).

Both the RNA- and the DNA-primed polymerase activities of the 8S and the 6S form of the enzyme coincided in the gradients shown in Fig. 4. Neither the 8S nor the 6S DNA polymerase had detectable endogenous template activities. Further, it was found when different fractions were mixed that the RNA-primed enzymatic activities of all fractions of the 8S DNA polymerase peak tested were 70–100% additive; the same was true when DNA-primed activities were measured. This suggests that no enhancing or inhibiting factor was present in this region of the gradient.

DISCUSSION

The distinctive RNase-sensitivity of the $s_{20,w}$ of the viral DNA-polymerase permitted a 40-fold purification of the enzyme based on the soluble radioactive protein of the virus. Since the particle weight of RSV is about 5×10^8, and its protein content is 60% (19), 1.5% at most of the mass of the virion can be DNA polymerase. This calculation assumes that the specific radioactivities of the enzyme and the structural proteins of the virus are the same. It follows that a maximum of 70 6S DNA polymerase molecules (110,000 daltons) may be present per virion. However, this is considered to be an upper estimate, because the 40-fold purified enzyme was contaminated by other structural proteins of the virus. The purified enzyme contained at least one protein component that had not previously been identified (10, 11) as a structural component of the virus. The enzyme also contained 10% of the soluble viral glycoprotein, which may not be an essential part of the polymerase because it consisted mainly of the two components of the 9S glycoprotein complex of the virus; the complex had no enzymatic activity.

Neither the 8S and the 6S DNA polymerase had endogenous template activities. This leaves open the question whether the reduction of the $s_{20,w}$ of the enzyme from 8S to 6S by RNase treatment is due to removal of short pieces of viral, or perhaps of cellular, RNA (20) without template activity. Such short pieces of viral RNA presumably arise by degradation of the 60–70S viral RNA (20) by virus-associated RNase (21), as tumor virus RNA is known to become RNase-sensitive in the presence of nonionic detergents (20). Short pieces of enzyme-associated RNA might enhance the activity of templates added to the enzyme. This is compatible with the decrease of enzymatic activity observed after RNase treatment.

The coincidence in sucrose gradients of both the RSV RNA- and the DNA-primed DNA polymerase activities, in both the 8S and the 6S form, makes it likely that the two activities reside in the same enzyme. This evidence does not exclude, however, that different sites on the enzyme or different factors might specify the RNA- or DNA-dependent activities. It would appear, then, that this enzyme, which is known to have rather nonspecific template requirements if primed by natural DNAs (4–8) or synthetic nucleic acids (4, 9), has specific template requirements for natural RNAs, i.e., preferential affinity for 60–70S RSV RNA. The finding that heat dissociation reduces the template activity of 60–70S RSV RNA to that of other natural RNAs suggests that the peculiar secondary or subunit structure of 60–70S RSV RNA (12, 18) may be essential for its template activity for the viral DNA polymerase.

63

NOTE ADDED IN PROOF

The soluble DNA polymerase was separated from more than 99% of the viral glycoprotein by chromatography on phosphocellulose.

We thank Dr. W. M. Stanley for encouragement and Drs. H. Rubin, G. S. Martin, M. Halpern, and M. Chamberlin for critical discussions. Marie O. Stanley rendered excellent assistance.

This investigation was supported by the United States Public Health Service research grant CA 11426 from the National Cancer Institute and by Cancer Research Funds of the University of California.

1. Temin, H. M., and S. Mizutani, *Nature*, **226**, 1211 (1970).
2. Baltimore, D., *Nature*, **226**, 1209 (1970).
3. Duesberg, P. H., and E. Canaani, *Virology*, **42**, 783 (1970).
4. Mizutani, S., D. Boettiger, and H. M. Temin, *Nature*, **228**, 424 (1970).
5. Spiegelman, S., A. Burny, M. R. Das, J. Keydar, J. Schlom, M. Travnicek, and K. Watson, *Nature*, **227**, 1029 (1970).
6. Riman, J., and G. S. Beaudreau, *Nature*, **228**, 427 (1970).
7. McDonnell, J. P., A-C. Garapin, W. E. Levinson, N. Quintrell, L. Fanshier, and M. O. Bishop, *Nature*, **228**, 433 (1970).
8. Fujinaga, K., J. T. Parsons, J. W. Beard, D. Beard, and M. Green, *Proc. Nat. Acad. Sci. USA*, **67**, 1432 (1970).
9. Spiegelman, S., A. Burny, M. R. Das, J. Keydar, J. Schlom, M. Travnicek, and K. Watson, *Nature*, **228**, 430 (1970).
10. Duesberg, P. H., H. L. Robinson, W. S. Robinson, R. J. Huebner, and H. C. Turner, *Virology*, **36**, 73 (1968).
11. Duesberg, P. H., G. S. Martin, and P. K. Vogt, *Virology*, **41**, 631 (1970).
12. Duesberg, P. H., and P. K. Vogt, *Proc. Nat. Acad. Sci. USA*, **67**, 1673 (1970).
13. Zillig, W., E. Fuchs, and R. L. Millette, in *Procedures in Nucleic Acid Research*, ed. G. L. Cantoni (Harper and Row, New York, 1966), p. 323.
14. Chamberlin, M., J. McGrath, and L. Waskell, *Nature*, **228**, 227 (1970); Knippers, R., *Nature*, **228**, 1050 (1970).
15. Martin, R. G., and B. N. Ames, *J. Biol. Chem.*, **236**, 1372 (1961).
16. *Handbook of Biochemistry*, ed. H. Sober (Chemical Rubber Company, Cleveland, Ohio, 1968), p. C-17.
17. Schachman, H. K., in *Ultracentrifugation in Biochemistry* (Academic Press, New York, 1959).
18. Duesberg, P. H., *Proc. Nat. Acad. Sci. USA*, **60**, 1511 (1968).
19. Vogt, P. K., *Advan. Virus Res.*, **11**, 293 (1965).
20. Duesberg, P. H., in *Current Topics in Microbiology and Immunology* (Springer-Verlag, New York, 1970), Vol. 51, p. 79.
21. Rosenbergova, M., F. Lacour, and J. Huppert, *C. R. Acad. Sci. Paris*, **260**, 5145 (1965).
22. Levinson, W., M. J. Bishop, N. Quintrell, and J. Jackson, *Nature*, **227**, 1023 (1970).

DNA of Rous Sarcoma Virus: Its Nature and Significance

Warren E. Levinson
Harold E. Varmus
Axel-Claude Garapin
J. Michael Bishop

The principal nucleic acids of the RNA tumor viruses (oncornaviruses) are a 70S single-stranded RNA (the putative viral genome) and two forms of low-molecular-weight RNA (*1*). Recently, however, small amounts of DNA have also been found in purified preparations of avian (*2, 3*) and murine (*4*) oncornaviruses. This observation is of interest in view of the substantial body of evidence indicating that DNA is es-

sential to both the replication of oncornaviruses and the induction of cellular transformation by these viruses (*5*). We now describe experiments designed to ascertain the source and significance of the DNA associated with virions of the Schmidt-Ruppin strain of Rous sarcoma virus (RSV).

Virus was propagated in secondary cultures of chick embryo fibroblasts, labeled with [³H]thymidine (14 c/

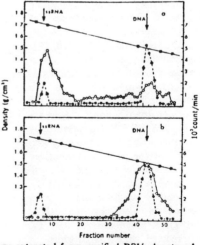

Fig. 1. Hybridization of DNA with RSV RNA. Denatured DNA (<0.1 μg) was incubated with 5 μg of 70S RSV RNA in 0.4 ml of annealing solution (*11*) for 24 hours at 37°C. The nucleic acids were then analyzed by equilibrium centrifugation in Cs₂SO₄ (*11*). *Escherichia coli* RNA and lambda phage DNA both labeled with ³²P served as density markers. (a) Virus-specific DNA synthesized by RNA-directed DNA polymerase. ³H-Labeled DNA was synthesized with the virion-associated polymerase of RSV (*7, 9*), and single-stranded DNA was isolated from the reaction product as described (*8*). This DNA is entirely complementary to RSV 70S RNA, and consequently can be extensively hybridized to viral RNA as illustrated here and reported (*11*). ●—●, ³²P, count/min; ○—○, ³H, count/min; ssRNA, single-stranded RNA marker; DNA, DNA marker. (b) Virion DNA. ³H-Labeled DNA was extracted from purified RSV, denatured with NaOH, and incubated with 70S RSV RNA as described above. The amount of virion DNA (< 0.1 μg) was estimated on the basis of the specific activity of DNA extracted from the cells used to produce the labeled virus. ●—●, ³²P, count/min; ○—○, ³H, count/min; ▣, density, g/cm³.

mmole), [^{14}C]uridine (55 mc/mmole), or [^{32}P]orthophosphate (all from Schwarz/Mann), and purified as described (2, 6). Nucleic acids were extracted from purified virus with sodium dodecyl sulfate and pronase (7), then fractionated by elution from hydroxyapatite (8). DNA comprises approximately 0.5 to 1.0 percent of the total nucleic acids obtained from RSV in this manner. Similar results were obtained with phenol extraction, although the recovery of nucleic acids was reduced (2).

The DNA extracted from purified RSV is double helical, as judged by its elution from hydroxyapatite (data not shown). The standards for this analysis were the single-stranded DNA of fd bacteriophage and the double-stranded DNA of avian cells [see (8) for details of the procedure and its standardization]. The RSV DNA is completely denatured to the single chain form when boiled in 3 mM EDTA for 10 minutes or when treated with 0.4N NaOH at 37°C for 1 hour (unpublished observation). These data indicate that virion DNA is composed of double-stranded molecules with no propensity to "snap back" after denaturation.

Virions of oncornaviruses contain an RNA-directed DNA polymerase (9) which transcribes the viral RNA genome into double-helical DNA (8, 10). It is conceivable that virion DNA represents the product of such transcription occurring within the virion. We tested this possibility by examining the ability of denatured virion DNA to anneal with 70S RSV RNA, purified by rate-zonal centrifugation in density gradients of sucrose (6). The annealed nucleic acids were analyzed by equilibrium centrifugation in Cs$_2$SO$_4$ (11). As a control, single-stranded DNA synthesized in vitro by the RNA-directed DNA polymerase of RSV (7, 8) was reacted with a large excess of 70S viral RNA (Fig. 1a). Virtually all of the DNA hybridizes with viral RNA, and consequently bands at approximately the same density as single-

stranded RNA. The nature and specificity of these hybrid structures have been recorded (11). No hybrids are formed when denatured virion DNA is reacted with 70S viral RNA (Fig. 1b). The breadth of the band of virion DNA is due to its low molecular weight [about 100,000 to 500,000; (2)] compared to that of the lambda bacteriophage DNA marker (about 30 × 10^6).

Failure of the virion DNA to hybridize with viral RNA under the above conditions could be ascribed to a more rapid interaction of complementary DNA strands to re-form double-helical molecules. We have tested this possibility with negative results. At the conclusion of the annealing reaction, the virion DNA still elutes from hydroxyapatite as single-stranded molecules (unpublished observation).

Having failed to find any complementarity between nucleotide sequences of virion DNA and viral RNA, we examined virion DNA for sequences homologous to those of cellular DNA. This was done by measuring the reassociation kinetics of various DNA's in the manner described by Britten and Kohne (12). As noted above, and illustrated further in Fig. 2a, denatured virion DNA does not reassociate at the concentrations now available. The incubation described in Fig. 2a was carried out in the presence of salmon sperm DNA, the reassociation of which proceeded normally. By contrast, denatured virion DNA does reanneal into a double-helical state when incubated in the presence of denatured avian cell DNA (Fig. 2b). Moreover, the extent of reassociation as a function of time is identical to that of the cellular DNA. We conclude that virion DNA of RSV shares extensive or complete sequence homology with the DNA of avian cells, and that populations of individual sequences are present in both types of DNA in about the same amount. Virion DNA of RSV is therefore probably derived in a random fashion from DNA of the avian host cell.

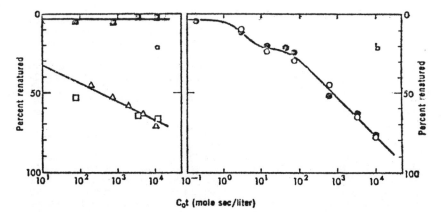

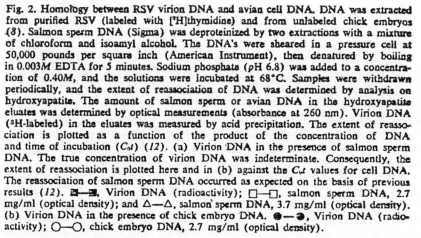

Cₒt (mole sec/liter)

Fig. 2. Homology between RSV virion DNA and avian cell DNA. DNA was extracted from purified RSV (labeled with [³H]thymidine) and from unlabeled chick embryos (8). Salmon sperm DNA (Sigma) was deproteinized by two extractions with a mixture of chloroform and isoamyl alcohol. The DNA's were sheared in a pressure cell at 50,000 pounds per square inch (American Instrument), then denatured by boiling in 0.003M EDTA for 5 minutes. Sodium phosphate (pH 6.8) was added to a concentration of 0.40M, and the solutions were incubated at 68°C. Samples were withdrawn periodically, and the extent of reassociation of DNA was determined by analysis on hydroxyapatite. The amount of salmon sperm or avian DNA in the hydroxyapatite eluates was determined by optical measurements (absorbance at 260 nm). Virion DNA (³H-labeled) in the eluates was measured by acid precipitation. The extent of reassociation is plotted as a function of the product of the concentration of DNA and time of incubation ($C_o t$) (12). (a) Virion DNA in the presence of salmon sperm DNA. The true concentration of virion DNA was indeterminate. Consequently, the extent of reassociation is plotted here and in (b) against the $C_o t$ values for cell DNA. The reassociation of salmon sperm DNA occurred as expected on the basis of previous results (12). ■—■, Virion DNA (radioactivity); □—□, salmon sperm DNA, 2.7 mg/ml (optical density); and △—△, salmon sperm DNA, 3.7 mg/ml (optical density). (b) Virion DNA in the presence of chick embryo DNA. ●—●, Virion DNA (radioactivity); ○—○, chick embryo DNA, 2.7 mg/ml (optical density).

Purified preparations of a number of DNA viruses contain virions that enclose host cell DNA rather than viral genome (13). These "pseudovirions" can generally be distinguished and purified by virtue of their unique buoyant densities. We have centrifuged RSV—doubly labeled with [³H]thymidine and [¹⁴C]uridine—to equilibrium in shallow density gradients of CsCl. There is no appreciable discrepancy between the densities of the particles containing DNA and RNA. However, the significance of this negative result is uncertain, because nucleic acids comprise only 1 to 2 percent of the total mass of RSV (1) and therefore contribute very little to the density of the virus particle.

At present, there is no evidence to suggest that virion DNA might be essential to the biological activity of RNA tumor viruses. We have examined this issue further by performing the following experiment. RSV-infected cells were exposed to bromodeoxyuridine (BUdR: 5 or 50 μg/ml) for 36 hours. Virus was harvested from these cells during the final 12 hours, purified, and tested for photosensitivity. Irradiation with visible light had no effect on its biological activity, which was measured by focus assay (14). The amount of BUdR and the dose of irradiation were similar to those used by Boettiger and Temin to photoinactivate infectious centers induced by RSV (15). The extent to which BUdR has sub-

67

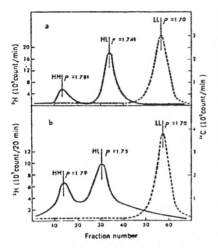

Fig. 3. Equilibrium centrifugation of BUdR-substituted DNA. RSV-infected cells were exposed to BUdR (5 μg/ml) for 24 hours, followed by a 12-hour exposure to both BUdR (5 μg/ml) and [³H]thymidine (50 μc/ml). At the conclusion of this 12-hour period, virus was harvested, and DNA was extracted from the cells (22). DNA was subsequently extracted from the purified virus in the same manner. Virion and cellular DNA were analyzed separately by equilibrium centrifugation in CsCl [40 rotor, 33,000 rev/min, 25°C, 60 hours; see (21)]. Normal avian DNA, labeled with [¹⁴C]thymidine, was included in both cases as a density marker (ρ = 1.70 g/cm³). The gradients were fractionated and samples were taken for determination of density and acid-precipitable radioactivity. LL, DNA containing two strands of normal density; HL, DNA containing one normal strand and one strand substituted with BUdR; HH, DNA containing both strands substituted with BUdR. (a) Cellular DNA. ——, ³H radioactivity (BUdR-substituted cellular DNA); – – –, ¹⁴C radioactivity (normal cellular DNA). (b) Virion DNA. ——, ³H radioactivity (BUdR-substituted virion DNA); – – –, ¹⁴C radioactivity (normal cellular DNA).

stituted for thymidine in virion DNA was determined by equilibrium centrifugation in CsCl (Fig. 3). The distributions of BUdR-substituted virion and cellular DNA's in these gradients are virtually identical. This observation supports our previous suggestion that virion DNA is derived from the normal pool of cellular DNA without special selection. The densities of the once-replicated (HL, ρ = 1.74–1.75) and twice-replicated (HH, ρ = 1.78–1.79) DNA's are indicative of maximum substitution by BUdR (16).

We conclude that the DNA associated with purified virions of RSV consists of a random sample of cellular DNA in a low-molecular-weight form. The possibility that the DNA is enclosed in "pseudovirions", rather than in biologically active virions, is still undetermined. However, the presence of small amounts of ribosomal RNA in RSV (1, 6) and other RNA tumor viruses (1) does point to the inclusion of normal cellular elements in virus preparations, either as adventitious contaminants or as virion constituents. A report that DNA is associated with the plasma membrane of human diploid cells (17) raises the possibility that the DNA found in oncornaviruses is an envelope constituent, acquired when virions are released from the host cell. Examination of purified viral nucleoids (18) for the presence of DNA should provide a test of this suggestion. Whatever its source, the virion DNA of RNA tumor viruses must be taken into account in any study of the RNA-directed DNA polymerase present in these viruses. We have evidence that as much as 5 to 10 percent of the total double-stranded DNA synthesized in vitro by enzyme-active virions consists of transcripts of the avian DNA associated with RSV virions. Other investigators have suggested that virion DNA might serve as the primer for initiation of RNA-directed synthesis within the virion (19), but more recent observations indicate that this function is served by a ribopolynucleotide (20). For the present, we consider the most reasonable conclusion to be that the DNA present in preparations of RSV is probably devoid of any special function in the life cycle of the virus.

68

References and Notes

1. W. S. Robinson and P. H. Duesberg, in *Molecular Basis of Virology*, H. Fraenkel-Conrat, Ed. (Reinhold, New York, 1968), p. 306; R. A. Bonar, L. Sverak, D. P. Bolognesi, A. J. Langlois, D. Beard, J. W. Beard, *Cancer Res.* 27, 1138 (1967); R. L. Erikson, *Virology* 37, 124 (1969); M. Travnicek, *Biochem. Biophys. Acta* 182, 427 (1969); J. M. Bishop, W. E. Levinson, D. Sullivan, L. Fanshier, N. Quintrell, J. Jackson, *Virology* 42, 805 (1970).
2. W. E. Levinson, J. M. Bishop, N. Quintrell, J. Jackson, *Nature* 227, 1023 (1970).
3. J. Riman and G. S. Beaudreau, *ibid.* 228, 427 (1970).
4. M. Rokutanda, H. Rokutanda, M. Green, K. Fujinaga, R. Kumar Ray, C. Gurgo, *ibid.* 227, 1026 (1970); N. Biswal, B. McCain, M. Benyesh-Melnick, *Virology*, in press.
5. H. M. Temin, in *The Biology of Large RNA Viruses*, R. D. Barry and B. W. J. Mahy, Eds. (Academic Press, London, 1970), p. 233.
6. J. M. Bishop, W. E. Levinson, D. Sullivan, L. Fanshier, N. Quintrell, J. Jackson, *Virology* 42, 182 (1970).
7. A. C. Garapin, J. P. McDonnell, W. Levinson, N. Quintrell, L. Fanshier, J. M. Bishop, *J. Virol.* 6, 589 (1970).
8. L. Fanshier, A. C. Garapin, J. McDonnell, A. Faras, W. Levinson, J. M. Bishop, *ibid.* 7, 77 (1971).
9. D. Baltimore, *Nature* 226, 1209 (1970); H. M. Temin and S. Mizutani, *ibid.*, p. 1211.
10. K. Fujinaga, J. T. Parsons, J. W. Beard, D. Beard, M. Green, *Proc. Nat. Acad. Sci. U.S.* 67, 1432 (1970); K. F. Manly, D. F. Smoler, E. Bromfeld, D. Baltimore, *J. Virol.* 7, 107 (1971).
11. S. Spiegelman, A. Burny, M. R. Das, J. Keydar, J. Schlom, M. Travnicek, K. Watson, *Nature* 227, 563 (1970); A. C. Garapin, L. Fanshier, J. Leong, J. Jackson, W. Levinson, J. M. Bishop, *J. Virol.* 7, 227 (1971).
12. R. J. Britten and D. E. Kohne, *Science* 161, 529 (1968).
13. M. R. Michel, B. Hirt, R. Weil, *Proc. Nat. Acad. Sci. U.S.* 58, 381 (1967); D. M. Trilling and D. Axelrod, *Science* 168, 268 (1970); A. J. Levine and A. K. Teresky, *J. Virol.* 5, 451 (1970).
14. W. Levinson, *Virology* 32, 74 (1967).
15. D. Boettiger and H. M. Temin, *Nature* 228, 622 (1970).
16. E. H. Simon, *Exp. Cell. Res.* 6 (Suppl.), 263 (1963).
17. R. H. Lerner, W. Mainke, D. A Goldstein, *Proc. Nat. Acad. Sci. U.S.* 63, 1212 (1971).
18. J. M. Coffin and H. M. Temin, *J. Virol.* 7, 625 (1971).
19. D. Baltimore and D. Smoler, *Proc. Nat. Acad. Sci. U.S.* 68, 1507 (1971).
20. I. M. Verma, E. Bromfeld, K. F. Manly, D. Baltimore, *Nature* 233, 131 (1971).
21. C. F. Brunk and V. Leick, *Biochim. Biophys. Acta* 179, 136 (1969).
22. E. H. Simon, *J. Mol. Biol.* 3, 101 (1961).
23. We thank L. Levintow for encouragement and support; N. Quintrell, J. Jackson, and R. Howard for technical assistance. Supported by PHS grants CA 12380, AI 08864, and AI 06362; NIH contract 71-2149; NIH training grant AI 00299; and the California Division of the American Cancer Society (ACS 556).

Deoxyribonucleic Acid Polymerase Associated with Avian Tumor Viruses: Secondary Structure of the Deoxyribonucleic Acid Product

LOIS FANSHIER, AXEL-CLAUDE GARAPIN, JEROME McDONNELL, ANTHONY FARAS, WARREN LEVINSON, AND J. MICHAEL BISHOP

A novel deoxyribonucleic acid (DNA) polymerase, which apparently transcribes DNA from a ribonucleic acid (RNA) template, has been discovered in association with the virions of RNA tumor viruses (1, 13). It has been suggested that the DNA synthesized by this enzyme serves as an intermediate in viral RNA replication, and that it is integrated into host DNA to provide for stable transformation (1, 12, 13). In view of these hypotheses, the precise nature of the enzymatic product is of substantial biological interest. Previous reports (6, 11) have established the fact that the enzyme initially synthesizes DNA:RNA hybrids. These are composed of nascent DNA chains hydrogen-bonded to molecules of their putative template, the 70S viral RNA. As the reaction progresses, DNA which is not associated with RNA also accumulates, eventually becoming the predominant product of enzymatic synthesis (6). On the presumption that this latter DNA may represent the biologically active form of enzymatic product, we have attempted to characterize its secondary structure by correlative analyses with equilibrium centrifugation and hydroxyapatite. We conclude that hybrid and nonhybrid DNA can be distinguished by use of a convenient batch-elution procedure with hydroxyapatite, and that the principal final product of the enzymatic reaction is double-stranded DNA. These studies have been performed with both the Schmidt-

Ruppin strain of Rous sarcoma virus (RSV) and avian myeloblastosis virus, with essentially identical results. Unless otherwise stated, the illustrated results pertain to RSV.

MATERIALS AND METHODS

Reagents. ^{3}H-thymidine triphosphate (^{3}H-TTP), 10 to 12 Ci/mmole, was obtained from Schwarz BioResearch, Inc., or New England Nuclear Corp.

Pancreatic ribonuclease A was obtained from Worthington Biochemical Corp. Stock solutions were boiled for 10 min to inactivate contaminating deoxyribonuclease.

Pronase (B grade) and the deoxyribonucleoside triphosphates deoxyadenosine, deoxycytidine, and deoxyguanosine triphosphate (dATP, dCTP, and dGTP) were obtained from Calbiochem.

Phenol (reagent grade) was from Mallinckrodt Chemical Works; hydroxyapatite (Bio-Gel HT), from Bio-Rad Laboratories, Richmond, Calif.; Nonidet-P 40 (NP-40), from Shell Chemical Co.; and Cs$_2$SO$_4$ (optical grade), from Gallard-Schlesinger.

Sodium phosphate buffer was used at pH 7.8, and concentrations were standardized by use of refractive index.

Propagation and purification of virus. RSV, Schmidt-Ruppin strain, and avian myeloblastosis virus were prepared as described previously (4, 6). The protein content of purified virus (generally 1.0 to 1.5 mg/ml) was determined by the method of Lowry et al. (7).

Enzyme reaction. DNA polymerase associated with

RSV was assayed as described previously (6). Standard reaction mixtures contained the following: 0.05 M tris(hydroxymethyl)aminomethane (Tris)-hydrochloride, pH 8.1; 0.01 M $MgCl_2$; 100 to 500 μg of viral protein per ml; 6×10^{-5} M dATP, dGTP, and dCTP; 2% β-mercaptoethanol (v/v); 10^{-6} to 5×10^{-6} M ^{3}H-TTP; and an appropriate concentration of NP-40, determined individually for each preparation of purified virus. As noted previously (6), the optimal concentration of detergent is apparently a function of the concentration of viral protein in the reaction mixture.

Preparation of enzymatic product. Nucleic acids were routinely extracted from reaction mixtures by the addition of sodium dodecyl sulfate (0.5%, w/v) and self-digested Pronase (500 μg/ml), followed by incubation at 37 C for 45 min and two phenol extractions at room temperature. When necessary, the nucleic acids were precipitated with ethyl alcohol; unlabeled HeLa cell RNA was used as carrier (4). On occasion, the phenol extraction was omitted and the nucleic acids were analyzed directly on hydroxyapatite after dilution of the sodium dodecyl sulfate to 0.025%. This variation has no apparent effect on the adsorption and elution properties of the nucleic acids.

Analysis of nucleic acid secondary structure with hydroxyapatite. Chromatography on hydroxyapatite provides a convenient means by which to ascertain the secondary structure of DNA (2, 3, 9). The following batch procedure was employed to facilitate the processing of relatively large numbers of samples. For present purposes, it provided essentially the same information as would column chromatography, but allowed the analysis of as many as 15 samples in a period of 3 to 4 hr. Commercially available hydroxyapatite proved entirely satisfactory for the procedure. Slight variations in the elution properties of DNA were noted among different lots of hydroxyapatite and sodium phosphate buffers, but this is of little consequence because appropriate nucleic acid standards were included in every batch of analyses. The capacity of hydroxyapatite used in these experiments was approximately 1 mg of nucleic acid per ml of packed volume.

Nucleic acids (minimum of 2,000 counts/min) were adsorbed to 0.5 ml (packed volume) of hydroxyapatite by shaking or mechanical agitation in conical centrifuge tubes at room temperature for 5 min. When possible, adsorption was performed in 0.01 M sodium phosphate. However, the presence of sodium chloride (0.2 M) and ethylenediaminetetraacetate (EDTA, 2×10^{-3} M) had no effect on either the adsorption or subsequent elution of nucleic acids.

Nucleic acids were eluted from the hydroxyapatite by successive washes (each 2 ml) with sodium phosphate solutions of increasing concentrations. A full elution series utilized 0.05 M steps from 0.05 to 0.3 M, with two separate washes at each step. The 0.05 M washes were performed at room temperature for 5 min; all subsequent washes were at 55 C for 8 min (10). The hydroxyapatite was kept in suspension by intermittent agitation with a Pasteur pipette. At the conclusion of each wash, the hydroxyapatite was sedimented by centrifugation at 2,000 rev/min (Sorvall

RC-3) for 1 min at room temperature. The clear supernatant was withdrawn, and the next sodium phosphate solution was added. Supernatants from each wash were analyzed for acid-precipitable radioactivity as described previously (4). The radioactivity eluted by the two washes at each concentration of phosphate was summed and expressed as the fraction of total radioactivity eluted by the entire series of washes. Recovery of nucleic acid (whether RNA, DNA, or DNA:RNA hybrid) was always greater than 90%.

Preparation of nucleic acid standards. The method used to isolate 70S RNA from purified RSV was described previously (4). DNA, labeled with ^{3}H-thymidine, was extracted from chick embryo fibroblasts according to the method of Martin (8), and was used without further fractionation. It contained double-stranded DNA with molecular weights of 10^7 to 3×10^7 daltons, as determined by the method of Burgi and Hershey (5); the native DNA (molecular weight, 2.8×10^7) of lambda phage was used as a sedimentation reference. ^{32}P-labeled lambda phage DNA and ^{3}H-labeled single-stranded DNA of fd phage (molecular weight, 2×10^6) were kindly provided by D. Roulland-Dussoix. The preparation of fd DNA used in these experiments had been largely converted from the native circular form to linear molecules by radioautolysis.

Analysis of nucleic acids by ultracentrifugation. Rate-zonal sedimentation through sucrose gradients and equilibrium centrifugation in Cs_2SO_4 have been described previously (6). Recoveries of nucleic acids from Cs_2SO_4 ranged between 50 and 90% provided that the gradients contained at least 0.001 M EDTA, that centrifugation was carried out in polyallomer tubes, and that optical-grade Cs_2SO_4 was used. We have observed no indication that the loss of nucleic acids in Cs_2SO_4 is in any manner selective with respect to DNA, RNA, and DNA:RNA hybrids.

RESULTS

Fractionation of single- and double-stranded DNA on hydroxyapatite: validation of the batch-elution procedure. The elution from hydroxyapatite of various single- and double-stranded DNA preparations is illustrated in Fig. 1. Native chick DNA eluted primarily in 0.25 M phosphate (Fig. 1a). If this eluate was recycled through a second series of adsorption and elutions, no DNA eluted prior to the 0.25 M phosphate wash. Thus, the small amount of DNA in the initial 0.1 to 0.15 M phosphate eluates (Fig. 1a) is probably single-stranded DNA rather than an artifact intrinsic to the adsorption-elution process. The effect of molecular weight on the elution of chick DNA was also examined. Native DNA, sheared to an average molecular weight of 10^6, eluted in a manner which is virtually identical to that of the unsheared DNA (Fig. 1b).

Denatured DNA of lambda phage (Fig. 1c) and chick fibroblasts (not illustrated) eluted

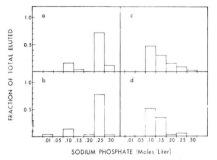

FIG. 1. *Fractionation of single- and double-stranded DNA on hydroxyapatite. DNA was prepared and analyzed on hydroxyapatite as described in Materials and Methods. (a) Native DNA from chick embryo fibroblasts, labeled with ³H-thymidine. Molecular weight of this DNA was approximately 10^7 to 3×10^7 daltons. (b) Native DNA from chick fibroblasts as in (a), but sheared by sonic treatment to an average molecular weight of 10^6 daltons. (c) ³²P-labeled DNA from lambda phage, denatured by boiling in 0.015 M NaCl-0.0015 M sodium citrate, pH 7, for 15 min, followed by quenching in an ice bath. (d) ³H-labeled single-stranded DNA from fd phage.*

predominantly in 0.1 to 0.15 M phosphate. The small amounts of DNA eluting in 0.2 and 0.25 M phosphate probably represent partially renatured material. On recycling of the 0.1 and 0.15 M eluates, no nucleic acid was found in any of the washes containing more than 0.15 M phosphate. The single-stranded DNA of fd phage eluted almost entirely in 0.1 to 0.15 M phosphate (Fig. 1d). Consequently, it is a more convenient and predictable standard for the procedure than are the denatured DNA preparations. We have not examined the effect of molecular topology on elution; therefore, to avoid any uncertainty in this regard, we deliberately chose fd DNA which was primarily linear (see Materials and Methods).

The results illustrated in Fig. 1 have proven to be consistent throughout the course of our investigation. Only relative variations have been observed: if double-stranded DNA elutes primarily in 0.3 M phosphate (rather than in 0.25 M, as in Fig. 1), single-stranded DNA will inevitably elute predominantly in 0.15 M phosphate rather than in the manner illustrated in Fig. 1. No appreciable elution of single-stranded DNA in phosphate concentrations greater than 0.15 M has ever been observed. These relative variations necessitate the inclusion of both single- and double-stranded DNA standards in every batch of analyses, but do not otherwise impair the reliability of the procedure.

Elution of DNA:RNA hybrid from hydroxyapatite. The initial product of DNA synthesis by the virion-associated polymerase is a DNA:RNA hybrid (6, 11), consisting of short, nascent DNA chains, hydrogen-bonded to viral RNA (6, 11; *in preparation*). This material is first detected as DNA which co-sediments with 70S viral RNA during rate-zonal centrifugation (6; also, see Fig. 8), and which has a buoyant density identical to that of single-stranded RNA (6, 11). Because the 70S DNA:RNA complex is a major constituent of early enzymatic product (6), it was mandatory to examine the elution of this material from hydroxyapatite prior to applying the batch-elution procedure to unfractionated product. Purified complex elutes from hydroxyapatite in a manner quite similar to that of isolated 70S viral RNA (Fig. 2a and b). We attribute this observation to the fact that each molecule of 70S DNA:RNA hybrid apparently contains a large segment of RNA which is not associated with DNA (6). Consequently, the hybrid possesses physicochemical properties similar to those of 70S viral RNA, i.e., similar sedimentation coefficient and buoyant density (6, 11), and similar elution from hydroxyapatite.

Treatment of the 70S complex with ribonuclease in 0.3 M NaCl produces a DNA:RNA hybrid with a low sedimentation velocity (ca. 4S; *in preparation*) and approximately equimolar contents of DNA and RNA as judged by buoyant density (6). Presumably, only the RNA which is directly hydrogen-bonded to DNA escapes hydrolysis by the ribonuclease (14). Hybrid treated in this manner eluted from hydroxyapatite in a manner similar but not identical to that of single-stranded DNA (Fig. 2c); the single-stranded DNA control in this assay was identical to that illustrated in Fig. 1d. Ribonuclease treatment in 3 mM EDTA, a condition which would be expected to hydrolyze even the hydrogen-bonded RNA (14), resulted in only a slightly greater proportion of DNA eluting in 0.1 M phosphate (Fig. 2d). We cannot presently explain the absence of a more distinctive difference between the elutions of the materials treated with ribonuclease in high and low concentrations of salt, but the matter is of no major consequence to our present purpose. The important fact is that ribonuclease treatment effectively removes all hybrid DNA from the region of double-stranded DNA elution. Thus, ribonuclease treatment prior to the hydroxyapatite assay should allow an unambiguous assessment of the amount of double-stranded DNA present in enzymatic product. The utility of this maneuver will be further illustrated below

Evolution of enzymatic product: correlative analysis with equilibrium centrifugation and

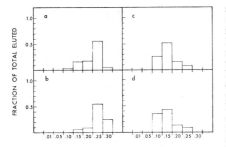

SODIUM PHOSPHATE (Moles Liter)

FIG. 2. *Elution of viral RNA and DNA : RNA hybrid from hydroxyapatite. ³²P-labeled 70S viral RNA was isolated from purified virus by phenol extraction and zonal centrifugation as described previously (4). DNA : RNA complex (70S) was prepared from a 1-hr enzymatic reaction. The product was extracted with sodium dodecyl sulfate-Pronase-phenol as described under Materials and Methods, and centrifuged through a 15 to 30% sucrose gradient containing 0.1 M NaCl-0.001 M EDTA-0.02 M Tris-hydrochloride, pH 7.4 (SW 65 rotor, 64,000 rev/min, 70 min, 4 C). The DNA co-sedimenting with 70S viral RNA was isolated from the gradient and stored frozen (−20 C) prior to analysis on hydroxyapatite. Adsorption to and elution from hydroxyapatite were not influenced by the presence of NaCl, EDTA, or sucrose. Appropriate control analyses were performed with single- and double-stranded DNA, but are not illustrated. The results were essentially as shown in Fig. 1. (a) ³H-labeled 70S DNA : RNA complex, synthesized by RSV-associated DNA polymerase. (b) ³²P-labeled 70S viral RNA. (c) 70S DNA : RNA complex, treated with ribonuclease (0.1 µg/ml) in 0.3 M NaCl at room temperature for 30 min. After ribonuclease treatment, the sample was adsorbed directly onto hydroxyapatite. Adsorption under identical conditions had no effect on the subsequent elution of single- and double-stranded DNA controls. (d) 70S DNA : RNA complex, treated with ribonuclease (10 µg/ml) in 3 mM EDTA at 37 C for 1 hr. Thereafter, the sample was adsorbed directly to hydroxyapatite. These conditions had no effect on the adsorption and elution of appropriate DNA controls.*

hydroxyapatite. We previously reported that the early product of enzymatic synthesis consists primarily of DNA:RNA hybrid, whereas the late product contains DNA which is not associated with RNA (6). Figure 3 illustrates a more detailed analysis of the progress of the enzymatic reaction, obtained by use of equilibrium centrifugation in Cs_2SO_4. After 15 min of synthesis (Fig. 3a), the product consisted almost exclusively of DNA which had a buoyant density virtually identical to that of single-stranded RNA. This observation conforms to our previous report that the initial product is a 70S DNA:RNA complex with the

same buoyant density as single-stranded RNA (6). The effect of ribonuclease treatment (in 0.3 M NaCl) on early (30 min) product is shown in Fig. 3b. The broad, symmetrical band with a mean density of 1.54 g/cc presumably represents the low-molecular-weight, equimolar hybrid of DNA:RNA obtained from the 70S complex as described above (Fig. 2). Hybrid material still predominated at 60 min (Fig. 3c), although there had been some reduction in the mean buoyant density. The latter change must reflect a decrease in the RNA-DNA ratio of the hybrid molecules, and could be due to lengthening of the nascent DNA chains or degradation by ribonuclease, or to a combination of these factors. We have data which indicate that there is considerable ribonuclease activity in the enzyme preparations under study in our laboratory (*in preparation*). Moreover, we presently have no evidence for the existence of other than short nascent DNA chains associated with viral RNA. Consequently, we must for the present ascribe all reductions in the buoyant density of hybrid product to degradative enzyme intrinsic to the reaction mixture.

After 4 hr of synthesis (Fig. 3d), the product consisted of two discrete populations, one banding in the DNA region of the density gradient (density ca. 1.45 g/cc) and the other corresponding to DNA:RNA hybrid (density ca. 1.54 g/cc). These data conform to our previous contention that at least two discrete enzymatic activities are operative (6, 7a), one producing the initial hybrid product and the other synthesizing nonhybrid DNA. However, the secondary structure of this latter DNA cannot be ascertained from its buoyant density, a fact which prompted the development and use of the hydroxyapatite assay.

Portions of the samples used in the equilibrium centrifugations illustrated by Fig. 3 were analyzed on hydroxyapatite (Fig. 4). Two primary conclusions can be drawn from these data. First, at no time did a significant proportion of the DNA elute in 0.1 M sodium phosphate. We therefore suggest that the product does not contain appreciable quantities of single-stranded DNA. The material which eluted in 0.15 M phosphate and which predominated early in the reaction must represent the hybrid molecules identified in equilibrium density gradients (Fig. 3a and c). The discrepancy between the elution pattern of this material and that of isolated 70S complex (Fig 2b) is probably due to partial degradation, as suggested by the results of equilibrium centrifugation (Fig. 3) and discussed above. Whatever the explanation of this discrepancy, it seems likely that the DNA eluting in 0.15 M phosphate represents (or has been derived from) hybrid structures, be-

73

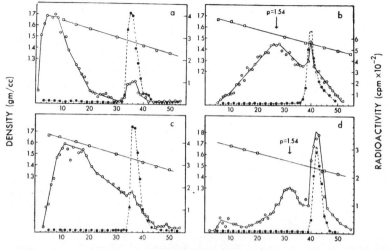

FRACTION NUMBER

FIG. 3. *Equilibrium centrifugation of enzymatic product from various time points. A standard reaction mixture containing 500 μg of viral protein, was prepared as described in Materials and Methods and incubated at 37 C At the various times, samples were withdrawn for extraction with sodium dodecyl sulfate-Pronase-phenol. Residua phenol was removed by three extractions with ether, and portions of each sample were analyzed by equilibrium centrifugation in Cs_2SO_4. ^{32}P-labeled lambda phage DNA was used as a density marker. (O) ^3H-labeled product; (●) ^{32}P-labeled lambda DNA. (a) Fifteen-minute product. (b) Thirty-minute product, treated with ribonuclease (0.1 μg/ml) in 0.3 M NaCl at room temperature for 30 min. Prior to centrifugation, the sample was re-extracted twice with phenol and three times with ether. (c) One-hour product. (d) Four-hour product.*

cause no other form of DNA is apparent in equilibrium density gradients until after 60 min (Fig. 3). [The small amount of product DNA found in the region of lambda DNA at early time points (Fig. 3a and b) is an occasional finding of uncertain significance. Note that in the series of analyses illustrated by Fig. 3 virtually none of this material is visible at 1 hr (Fig. 3c). Both denatured lambda DNA and denatured enzymatic product band at approximately 1.48 g/cc in these gradients.] Second, appreciable quantities of double-stranded DNA (eluting in 0.25 M phosphate) began to appear at about 2 hr. At 4 hr, over 30% of the total product eluted in 0.25 M phosphate (Fig. 4f). By comparison with the results of equilibrium centrifugation (Fig. 3d), we conclude that the DNA banding at a density of approximately 1.45 g/cc consists mainly of double-stranded molecules. This issue will be examined further below.

Time course of accumulation of double-stranded DNA: use of a modified hydroxyapatite assay. After treatment with ribonuclease, the elution of the DNA:RNA hybrid enzymatic product from hydroxyapatite no longer overlapped that of

double-stranded DNA (Fig. 2). This observation, and the fact that double-stranded DNA eluted almost entirely in 0.25 to 0.3 M phosphate, allowed a convenient abbreviation of the hydroxyapatite assay. Samples of nucleic acid were treated with ribonuclease in low concentrations of salt (usually 3 mM EDTA), and then adsorbed directly onto hydroxyapatite. Elutions were performed with 0.05, 0.20, and 0.30 M phosphate. Material eluting in 0.2 M phosphate was considered to be hybrid or single-stranded DNA, or both (Fig. 5a and c), whereas the 0.3 M phosphate eluate contained essentially all of the double-stranded DNA (Fig. 5b). The procedure does not discriminate between hybrid molecules and single-stranded DNA, but this is of no consequence because the product apparently contains insignificant amounts of single-stranded DNA (Fig. 4). Figures 5d–h illustrate the use of this procedure to analyze the accumulation of enzymatic products. Hybrid DNA (eluting in 0.2 M phosphate) was the exclusive product until approximately 2 hr, after which double-stranded DNA accumulated steadily. Late enzymatic

74

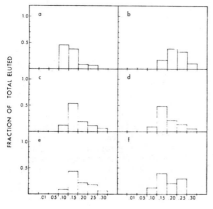

FIG. 4. *Analysis of enzymatic product on hydroxy-apatite. Portions of the samples prepared as described in Fig. 3 were analyzed on hydroxyapatite. Controls included single-stranded fd DNA, the 70S DNA:RNA complex isolated as described for Fig. 2, and double-stranded DNA (the last is not illustrated; the results were identical to those shown in Fig. 1). None of the samples was treated with ribonuclease. (a) Single-stranded DNA of fd phage; (b) 70S DNA:RNA complex; (c) 30-min product; (d) 1-hr product; (e) -hr product; (f) 4-hr product.*

product was at least 70% double-stranded DNA (Fig. 5h), a more detailed analysis of which is presented below.

Final product of the enzymatic reaction is double-stranded DNA. After 12 hr of enzymatic synthesis, no hybrid molecules were detectable in the product by equilibrium centrifugation (Fig. 6a). Analysis of this late DNA on hydroxyapatite is illustrated in Fig. 7. The bulk (70%) of the material eluted in 0.25 M phosphate, in contrast to the double-stranded DNA control, a major portion of which eluted in 0.3 M phosphate in this particular assay (Fig. 7b). We attribute this difference to the extremely low molecular weight of the DNA product (6; also, see Fig. 8). Ribonuclease treatment had no effect on the elution pattern (Fig. 7d), a fact which indicates that hybrid material was not contributing to the nucleic acid eluted in 0.25 M phosphate. Denaturation of late product with either heat or alkali caused it to elute as single-stranded DNA (see Fig. 1d and 4a). We conclude that the final enzymatic product consists primarily of double-stranded DNA, the synthesis of which is initiated subsequent to the production of significant quantities of DNA:RNA hybrid.

Analysis of low-molecular-weight enzymatic product on hydroxyapatite. In addition to the 70S DNA:RNA complex described above, prolonged enzymatic reactions produced low-molecular-weight DNA with sedimentation coefficients of 4

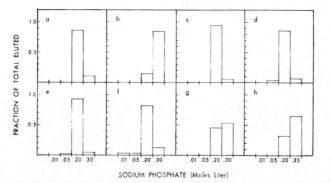

FIG. 5. *Abbreviated hydroxyapatite analysis of enzymatic product. Samples of a standard enzymatic reaction were extracted at various time points as described for Fig. 3. Small portions of these were diluted into 3 mM EDTA (maximum NaCl concentration, 0.01 M after dilution) and treated with ribonuclease (10 μg/ml) for 1 hr at 37 C prior to analysis on hydroxyapatite. All controls were treated with ribonuclease in the same manner. Nucleic acids were eluted from hydroxyapatite with successive washes of 0.05, 0.20, and 0.30 M sodium phosphate as described under Materials and Methods. (a) Single-stranded fd DNA; (b) double-stranded chick DNA; (c) 70S DNA:RNA complex, purified as described for Fig. 2; (d) 30-min product; (e) 1-hr product; (f) 2-hr product; (g) 4-hr product; (h) 12-hr product.*

75

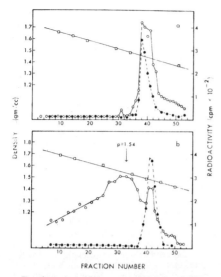

FIG. 6. *Analysis of enzymatic product by equilibrium centrifugation in Cs_2SO_4. (a) Avian myeloblastosis virus, 12-hr product. Nucleic acids were extracted from a standard reaction mixture [supplemented with phosphoenol pyruvate and pyruvate kinase (6)] after 12 hr of incubation. The energy-generating system has no effect on the nature of the product at any point in the reaction, but prolongs enzymatic activity by a factor of at least two (6). The nucleic acids were centrifuged to equilibrium in Cs_2SO_4, with ^{32}P-labeled lambda phage DNA as a density marker. (○) ^3H-labeled product; (●) ^{32}P-labeled lambda DNA. (b) Low-molecular-weight product at 1 hr. Nucleic acids were extracted from a standard reaction mixture at 1 hr, precipitated with ethyl alcohol, and separated into 70S complex and low-molecular-weight DNA by rate-zonal centrifugation through a 15 to 30% sucrose gradient (see Fig. 8). The DNA sedimenting at approximately 4 to 15S was recovered from the gradient and analyzed by equilibrium centrifugation in Cs_2SO_4. ^{32}P-labeled lambda phage DNA was used as a density marker. (○) ^3H-labeled product; (●) ^{32}P-labeled lambda DNA.*

to 15S (Fig. 8; also *in preparation*). As the reaction proceeded, the accumulation of low-molecular-weight DNA surpassed that of 70S complex, so that the former became the predominant enzymatic product by 2 hr (Fig. 8 and 9). Analyses with equilibrium centrifugation (Fig. 6b) and hydroxyapatite (Fig. 10 and 11) indicated that the low-molecular-weight material isolated by zonal centrifugation is composed of both double-stranded DNA and substantial amounts

of hybrid. In fact, a sample taken at 30 min contained virtually no double-stranded DNA (Fig. 10a). As the reaction progressed, double-stranded DNA accumulated in a manner similar to that illustrated in Fig. 5. At early time points, the low-molecular-weight population generally contained proportionately more double-stranded DNA than did the unfractionated product (compare Fig. 10b and c to Fig. 5e and f) because of the absence of 70S hybrid from the isolated low-molecular-weight DNA. Nevertheless, DNA:RNA hybrids were present in the low-molecular-weight population, as indicated by the elution of radioactivity in 0.15 and 0.20 M phosphate, and by the fact that the elution profile changed after ribonuclease treatment (Fig. 11), with an increase in the DNA eluting in 0.10 to 0.15 M phosphate and a concomitant decrease in the amount of DNA in the 0.20 M eluate.

DISCUSSION

The exact function of the DNA polymerase associated with RNA tumor viruses has yet to be established, but it is generally assumed that some or all of the DNA synthesized by this enzyme becomes integrated into host DNA in order to provide for stable transformation (12). If this be the case, then the secondary structure of the final enzymatic product is of crucial importance because it would determine the mechanism by which integration is accomplished. For example,

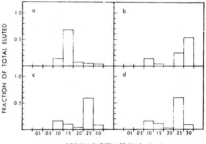

FIG. 7. *Analysis of 12-hr enzymatic product on hydroxyapatite. A portion of the 12-hr product (avian myeloblastosis virus) used for the equilibrium centrifugation illustrated in Fig. 6a was analyzed on hydroxyapatite. (a) Single-stranded fd phage DNA; (b) double-stranded chick DNA; (c) 12-hr enzymatic product; (d) 12-hr enzymatic product, treated with ribonuclease. A sample of the extracted product was diluted into 3 mM EDTA and treated with ribonuclease (10 μg/ml, 1 hr, 37 C) prior to analysis on hydroxyapatite.*

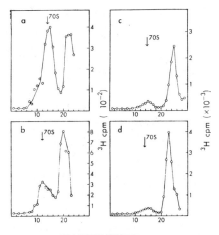

FRACTION NUMBER

FIG. 8. *Zonal centrifugation of enzymatic product. Nucleic acids were extracted from a standard reaction mixture (containing 500 µg of viral protein) at various time points, precipitated with ethyl alcohol, and sedimented through gradients of 15 to 30% sucrose containing 0.1 M NaCl-0.001 M EDTA-0.02 M Tris-hydrochloride, pH 7.4 (SW 65 rotor, 60,000 rev/min, 70 min, 4 C). Gradient fractions were analyzed for acid precipitable radioactivity as described previously (6). The rapidly sedimenting DNA has previously been identified as a hydrogen-bonded complex of nascent DNA and viral RNA (6). The slowly sedimenting population (4 to 15S) was recovered from the gradients for further analysis (Fig. 6b and 10). ^{32}P-labeled 70S RSV RNA was used as a sedimentation marker. (a) Thirty-minute product. (b) One-hour product. (c) Two-hour product. (d) Four-hour product.*

a double-stranded product might require no further biochemical modification prior to integration by normal mechanisms of recombination. The potential biological significance of this issue prompted us to examine the secondary structure of polymerase product in some detail. Our data indicate that the principal final product of the enzymatic reaction (in the case of RSV and avian myeloblastosis virus) is double-stranded DNA. Appreciable amounts of single-stranded DNA could not be detected at any point during the course of the reaction, although the data in this regard are not decisive.

Synthesis of double-stranded DNA is preceded by the synthesis of DNA:RNA hybrids which presumably represent intermediates in the enzymatic reaction. The precise mechanism by which double-stranded DNA is synthesized has not yet been elucidated, but we have shown that the

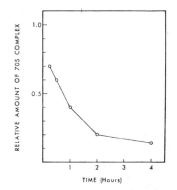

FIG. 9. *Proportions of 70S DNA:RNA complex and low-molecular-weight DNA at various time points in the polymerase reaction. Enzymatic product from various time points was analyzed by zonal centrifugation as in Fig. 8. The radioactivity contained in the 70S peak and that in the low-molecular-weight population were summed, and the ratio of the two was computed for each time point. The change in ratio as the reaction progresses is not due simply to cessation of the production of 70S complex, because there is an absolute increase in the latter for at least 2 to 3 hr (unpublished observations of the authors).*

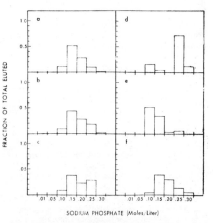

SODIUM PHOSPHATE (Moles/Liter)

FIG. 10. *Analysis of low-molecular-weight product on hydroxyapatite. DNA sedimenting at approximately 4 to 15S was recovered from sucrose gradients similar to those illustrated in Fig. 8 and analyzed on hydroxyapatite. (a) Thirty-minute product. (b) One-hour product. (c) Two-hour product. (d) Double-stranded chick DNA. (e) Single-stranded fd DNA. (f) 70S DNA:RNA complex, prepared as described for Fig. 2.*

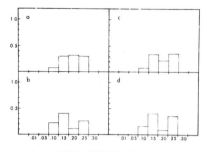

Fig. 11. *Analysis of ribonuclease-treated low-molecular-weight product on hydroxyapatite. DNA sedimenting at approximately 4 to 15S was recovered from sucrose gradients similar to those illustrated in Fig. 8, and was analyzed on hydroxyapatite before and after treatment with ribonuclease (10 μg/ml, 3 mM EDTA, 1 hr, 37 C). (a) Two-hour product, control. (b) Two-hour product, ribonuclease-treated. (c) Four-hour product, control. (d) Four-hour product, ribonuclease-treated.*

responsible enzyme can be inhibited by actinomycin D, and that it is capable of using exogenous DNA (either single- or double-stranded) as template (7a; *unpublished data*). In the absence of exogenous template, the synthesis of double-stranded DNA is totally dependent upon the synthesis of DNA:RNA hybrid. Thus, if synthesis of the latter is inhibited by treatment of the enzyme complex with ribonuclease prior to initiation of the reaction, the synthesis of double-stranded DNA is also inhibited (7a).

The initial product of the enzymatic reaction is a hydrogen-bonded complex of nascent DNA and viral RNA, with a sedimentation coefficient of approximately 70S (6). As the reaction progresses, substantial amounts of slowly sedimenting (4 to 15S) DNA:RNA hybrids accumulate (Fig. 10). This material contains only short (ca. 4S) chains of DNA (*in preparation*), and, for the present, we must assume that it is derived from the 70S hybrids by the degradative action of ribonuclease which is intrinsic to the virion-enzyme complex (*in preparation*). We have yet to determine whether or not these low-molecular-weight hybrids are active as templates for the synthesis of double-stranded DNA.

In its native state, the 70S hybrid cannot be reliably differentiated from double-stranded DNA by analysis on hydroxyapatite (Fig. 2). This observation is at variance with previous reports which described the successful resolution of DNA:RNA hybrids from both single- and

double-stranded DNA by chromatography on hydroxyapatite (10). We ascribe this discrepancy to the fact that the 70S hybrid contains a very small proportion of DNA, and the nature of its elution is therefore determined by the RNA constituent. Consequently, the intact hybrid molecule elutes in a manner quite similar to that of isolated 70S viral RNA (Fig. 2). As expected, partial or complete degradation of the RNA constituent substantially alters the elution of the hybrid (Fig. 2 and 10). This fact facilitates an unambiguous analysis of reaction product for the presence of double-stranded DNA, and should facilitate the use of the hydroxyapatite procedure in experiments designed to detect a precursor-product relationship between hybrid molecules and double-stranded DNA.

ACKNOWLEDGMENTS

We are indebted to Nancy Quintrell, Barbara Evans, and Jean Jackson for assistance, to D. Roulland-Dussoix for gifts of DNA extracted from purified lambda and fd phages, and to Leon Levintow for his support, encouragement, and editorial assistance.

This work was supported by Public Health Service grants AI 06862 and AI 08864 from the National Institute of Allergy and Infectious Diseases, by a grant from the California Division of the American Cancer Society (#483), and by the Cancer Research Coordinating Committee of the University of California.

LITERATURE CITED

1. Baltimore, D. 1970. RNA-dependent DNA polymerase in virions of RNA tumour viruses. Nature (London) 226: 1209–1211.
2. Bernardi, G. 1969. Chromatography of nucleic acids on hydroxyapatite. I. Chromatography of native DNA. Biochim. Biophys. Acta 174:423–434.
3. Bernardi, G. 1969. Chromatography of nucleic acids on hydroxyapatite. II. Chromatography of denatured DNA. Biochim. Biophys. Acta 174:435–448.
4. Bishop, J. M., W. E. Levinson, N. Quintrell, L. Fanshier, and J. Jackson. 1970. The low molecular weight RNA's of Rous sarcoma virus. I. The 4S RNA. Virology 42:182–195.
5. Burgi, E., and A. D. Hershey. 1963. Sedimentation rate as a measure of molecular weight of DNA. Biophys. J. 3:309.
6. Garapin, A.-C., J. P. McDonnell, W. Levinson, N. Quintrell, L. Fanshier, and J. M. Bishop. 1970. Deoxyribonucleic acid polymerase associated with Rous sarcoma virus and avian myeloblastosis virus: properties of the enzyme and its product. J. Virol. 6:589–598.
7. Lowry, O. H., N. J. Rosebrough, A. L. Farr, and R. J. Randall. 1951. Protein measurement with the Folin phenol reagent. J. Biol. Chem. 193:265–275.
7a. McDonnell, J. P., A.-C. Garapin, W. E. Levinson, N. Quintrell, L. Fanshier, and J. M. Bishop. 1970. DNA polymerase associated with Rous sarcoma virus: delineation of two reactions with actinomycin. Nature 228: 433–435.
8. Martin, M. A. 1969. Characteristics of the Syrian hamster ribonucleic acid present in cells transformed by polyoma, simian virus 40, or adenovirus 12. J. Virol. 3:119–125.
9. Miyazawa, Y., and C. A. Thomas, Jr. 1965. Nucleotide composition of short segments of DNA molecules. J. Mol. Biol. 11:223–237.
10. Siebke, J. C., and T. Ekren. 1970. Chromatography of RNA-DNA complexes on hydroxyapatite. A method for the separation of complementary strands in T2 DNA. Eur. J. Biochem. 12:380–386.

78

11. Spiegelman, S., A. Burny, M. B. Das, J. Keydar, J. Schlom, M. Travnicek, and K. Watson. 1970. Characterization of the products of RNA-directed DNA polymerases in oncogenic RNA viruses. Nature (London) 227:563–567.

12. Temin, H. M. 1964. Homology between RNA from Rous sarcoma virus and DNA from Rous sarcoma virus-infected cells. Proc. Nat. Acad. Sci. U.S.A. 52:323–329.

13. Temin, H. M., and S. Mizutani. 1970. RNA-dependent DNA polymerase in virions of Rous sarcoma virus. Nature (London) 226:1211–1213.

14. Warner, R. C., H. H. Samuels, M. J. Abbot, and J. S. Krakow. 1963. Ribonucleic acid polymerase of Azobacter vinelandii. II. Formation of DNA-RNA hybrids with single-stranded DNA as primer. Proc. Nat. Acad. Sci. U.S.A. 49:533–538.

GENETIC VARIANTS

JOHN P. BADER
NANCY R. BROWN

Induction of Mutations in an RNA Tumour Virus by an Analogue of a DNA Precursor

IF the replication of RNA tumour viruses involves a DNA replicative intermediate[1-3], precursor analogues which modify DNA could inactivate the viral progeny by causing occasional errors in base pairing during transcription of RNA from DNA. Each RNA molecule transcribed might be defective in certain genes, but because different molecules would carry different defects, there would be intracellular complementarity. Nonetheless, incorporation of individual RNA molecules into virions would give defective particles. Such defective particles have been found after infection of cells by Rous sarcoma virus (RSV) and exposure of these cells to 5-bromodeoxyuridine (BrdU)[4], an analogue of deoxythymidine. An extension of these studies is described here. The RSV stock consisted of transforming Bryan RSV_0, the non-transforming Rous associated virus (RAV), and phenotypic mixtures.

The timing of the addition of BrdU was critical to its effect on RSV; infectivity was decreased only if BrdU was present during the first 12 h immediately after exposure of cells to virus (Table 1). Exposure of cells to BrdU for 12 h before infection or 12 h after infection produced no decrease in the yield of infectious virus.

Because mutants of avian sarcoma viruses can be obtained which fail to transform cells at high temperature[6,7] we examined the yields of virus from BrdU-treated cultures for temperature sensitive mutants. The RSV produced by cells exposed to BrdU immediately after infection was examined for the ability to transform cells at 36° C and at 40.5° C. Initially plates were placed at the respective temperatures immediately after addition of virus, but cells grew slowly at 36° C and the efficiency of infection by control RSV was only 50% of that at 40.5° C (Table 2). In all later experiments, plates were incubated at 40.5° C for 2 or 3 days after infection, then half were transferred to 36° C.

The numbers of foci induced by control RSV stocks at 36° C never exceeded those at 40.5° C; usually less foci were found at the lower temperature even when incubated first at 40.5° C (Table 2). But when plates receiving BrdU–RSV were transferred from 40.5° C to 36° C there was a substantial increase in the number of foci that was particularly apparent

Table 1 Effect of BrdU on Infectious Virus Production of Freshly Infected Cells

BrdU μg/ml.	Interval of exposure to BrdU (h)		
	−12 to 0	0.5 to 12	12 to 24
	(f.f.u. test/f.f.u. control)		
None	1.0	1.0	1.0
100	1.5	0.03	0.93
50	1.8	0.14	1.1
25	2.6	0.25	0.78

Cells from individual chick embryos were propagated in growth medium—Eagle's MEM with additional glucose (2 g/l. final conc.), sodium pyruvate (5 mM), penicillin (50 U/ml.), streptomycin (50 μg/ml.), 10% tryptose phosphate broth, and 5 or 10% foetal bovine serum. A clonal isolate of Rous sarcoma virus$_0$ (Bryan "high titre") containing Rous associated virus$_1$ was propagated and used as Rous sarcoma virus (RSV) stock. Sparse secondary cultures of cells were exposed to BrdU for a 12 h interval just before, immediately after, or 12 h after exposure of cells to RSV, five focus-forming units (f.f.u.) per cell. Cell culture fluids were collected 24 h after infection and subsequently assayed by the focus forming method[5].

when the plates were compared with those with control virus. In several experiments, the comparative efficiency of transformation at 36° C by BrdU–RSV ranged between 1.3 and 1.9 times that of control RSV (Table 2). Also, direct incubation

Table 2 Effect of BrdU Treatment on Transformation Efficiency at 40.5° C and 36° C

	Temperature of incubation			40.5→ 36° C/ 40.5° C	36° C/ 40.5° C
	40.5° C	40.5°→36° C	36° C		
Control	2,328 * (24) †	1,654 (24)	560 (12)	0.71	0.49
BrdU	2,475 (36)	3,344 (36)	840 (18)	1.35	0.70
BrdU/ control	—	—	—	1.9	1.4

Chick embryo cells were exposed to BrdU (100 μg/ml.) for 12 h immediately after infection with RSV; the BrdU-containing medium was then replaced with growth medium. These fluids, and others from cultures without BrdU, were collected 24 h after infection. After a preliminary titration, diluted samples (25–200 f.f.u. at 40.5° C) were added to chick embryo cells as in a standard focus assay. Equivalent plates were incubated (1) 6 days at 40.5° C, (2) 2 days at 40.5° C and switched to 36° C for an additional 5 days, or (3) only at 36° C for 10 days. The ratios were calculated from the average number of foci per plate.

* Total foci counted.

† Total plates.

Table 3 Transformation by RSV from BrdU-treated Cells

Cultures with added BrdU	Temperature of incubation		
	40.5° C	40.5°→36° C	40.5°→36° C/ 40.5° C
Newly infected	485 (8)	632 (8)	1.3
Established infected	712 (8)	631 (8)	0.89
BrdU pretreated then infected without BrdU	635 (8)	540 (8)	0.85

Cells infected by RSV 7 days earlier and transferred twice (established infected cultures) and newly infected cells were exposed to BrdU for 12 h. The medium was then replaced with complete growth medium. Another group of cultures was exposed to BrdU for 24 h before infection with RSV in the absence of BrdU. Culture fluids were collected 24 h after infection and diluted to give 25–150 foci per plate at 40.5° C.

at 36° C immediately after infection produced a greater decrease in control RSV foci than in BrdU–RSV foci. Again the comparative efficiency of BrdU–RSV at the lower temperature was 1.2 to 1.8 times higher than control RSV in several experiments. In one experiment cultures were shifted from 36° C to 40.5° C after 3 days of incubation and compared with cultures kept permanently at 36° C. Although the number of foci increased slightly at the higher temperature in both groups, the comparative increase was 1.2 times greater with control RSV.

These results suggest that a significant proportion of the virions produced by BrdU-treated cells contain a genetic defect (or defects) which cause a sensitivity of the transformation process to increased temperature. Established virus-producing cells treated with BrdU did not produce such temperature-sensitive populations, nor did cells pretreated with BrdU before infection (Table 3). Also, the comparative difference in transformation efficiencies at high and low temperatures diminished in culture fluids collected 30, 36 and 48 h after infection and BrdU treatment, and after 48 h differences between BrdU–RSV and control RSV were undetectable. In other words, with increasing time after infection of cells and exposure to BrdU, temperature-sensitive transforming virions became a decreasing proportion of the general virion population.

Attempts were made to isolate RSV defective in the genomic region responsible for transformation. Selection was made for the production of virus 40.5° C which was infectious for chick embryo cells and which later transformed cells at 36° C but not at 40.5° C. Virus-producing cells therefore were producing Rous associated virus$_1$ (RAV$_1$), as well as

Table 4 Isolation of RSV Mutants Temperature-sensitive for Transformation

No. of foci on original plate	Total clones	Total temperature-sensitive
BrdU–RSV > 25	79	9
BrdU–RSV < 10	26	6
BrdU–RSV 1 or 2	14	5
Control RSV > 25	27	0
Control RSV < 10	15	0

Cells were infected with BrdU–RSV or control RSV and overlaid with a nutrient agar medium containing 1% turkey anti-RSV (Bryan "high titre") serum. Foci developing at 36° C were observed microscopically and isolated by adding a small amount of liquid medium, scraping the area of the focus, and drawing the cells into a Pasteur pipette. The cells were propagated at 40.5° C in 35 mm plastic Petri dishes until suitable populations for testing were obtained. Culture fluids were collected and examined for ability to transform cells at 36° and 40.5° C.

temperature-sensitive Rous sarcoma virus$_0$ (RSV$_0$) (transformed cells without RAV$_1$ have been isolated also, but are inadequately characterized and are not considered here).

Of 119 transformed clones from foci induced by BrdU–RSV, twenty yielded RSV which failed to induce transformation at 40.5° C (Table 4). Of these, seven clones produced RSV which transformed cells only at the lower temperature, while cells seemed essentially normal at 40.5° C. The other thirteen clones produced virus which also altered the morphology of cells at 40.5° C but only when infection was made using high multiplicities of virus per cell. The morphological changes appearing in these conditions were atypical of the transformation characteristic of the Bryan "high titre" strain of RSV. This phenomenon could be a result of a partially defective product of an altered viral gene. The mutants can be considered "leaky". No temperature-sensitive RSV was found in clonal isolates of foci induced by control RSV (Table 4).

The production of mutations in RSV by BrdU demonstrates that the replicative form of the virus, at least the region determining transformation, is DNA. Radioactive BrdU is not incorporated into RNA in chick embryo cells[4]. Also, BrdU fails to affect the infectivity of other non-oncogenic RNA viruses[8], or even RSV in established infected cells, where the requirement for DNA synthesis has been fulfilled. Furthermore, no temperature-sensitivity was found in RSV populations derived from established infected cultures exposed to BrdU, or in virus derived from cells treated with BrdU prior to infection.

The occurrence of RNA-dependent DNA polymerase in RNA tumour virions[9,10] provides biochemical evidence that a viral DNA could be the replicative form. Some genetic evidence had also been obtained, for defective particles have been produced by BrdU treatment[4]. The experiments reported here provide further genetic evidence that a gene contained in viral RNA is transcribed from DNA.

The mechanism of selection of these mutants restricted the defect to the gene or genes determining transformation. Other genes of RSV_0 may be affected in any single isolate, but these defects, if present, are complemented by the concomitant production of RAV_1, which would provide enzymes and structural proteins for the production of infectious RSV virions. The production of fully infectious virus at the higher temperature (40.5° C) shows that there is no interference with the production and packaging of viral RNA, an observation similar to that described by Martin[7]. This demonstrates that the temperature-sensitive element required for transformation is a gene product, rather than interference with viral RNA synthesis. Attempts to identify this product are under investigation in this laboratory.

[1] Bader, J. P., *Mono. Nat. Cancer Inst.*, **17**, 781 (1964).
[2] Temin, H. M., *Mono. Nat. Cancer Inst.*, **17**, 557 (1964).
[3] Bader, J. P., in *The Biochemistry of Viruses* (edit. by Levy, H. B.) (Dekker, New York, 1969).
[4] Bader, J. P., and Bader, A. V., *Proc. US Nat. Acad. Sci.*, **67**, 843 (1970).
[5] Temin, H. M., and Rubin, H., *Virology*, **6**, 669 (1958).
[6] Toyoshima, K., and Vogt, P. K., *Virology*, **39**, 930 (1969).
[7] Martin, G. S., *Nature*, **227**, 1021 (1970).
[8] Bader, J. P., *Virology*, **22**, 462 (1964).
[9] Baltimore, D., *Nature*, **226**, 1209 (1970).
[10] Temin, H. M., and Mizutani, S., *Nature*, **226**, 1211 (1970).

A Mutant of Rous Sarcoma Virus (Type O) Causing Fusiform Cell Transformation[1] (35039)

SAIJI YOSHII AND PETER K. VOGT

The interaction between Rous sarcoma virus (RSV) and cell is determined by viral phenotype and genotype. The best studied phenotypic properties of RSV are those belonging to the viral envelope. They affect viral host range, sensitivity to interference with avian leukosis viruses and interaction with neutralizing antibody. On the other hand, cellular transformation appears to be dependent on expression of the viral genome. In the course of transformation the virus influences cellular morphology as well as social behavior, and various genetic strains of RSV differ in their modification of host cell properties (1–4). The most conspicuous of these differences is that between RSV which causes the transformed cells to become spherical and RSV which bestows a fusiform shape on the cell.

The Bryan high-titer strain of RSV commonly occurs in the form of pseudotypes which are the result of excessive phenotypic mixing with avian leukosis viruses (5). From such pseudotype stocks an RSV has been derived which causes round cell transformation and no longer contains overt avian leukosis viruses (6, 7). This agent is known as RSV type O. An agent inducing exclusively fusiform cell transformation was also derived from the Bryan high-titer strain of RSV (1, 2). Available preparations of this fusiform

RSV are likely to consist of pseudotype virus because they also contain high titers of non-transforming avian leukosis viruses. Therefore, it was suspected that the true nature of fusiform RSV had been obscured by phenotypic mixing with avian leukosis viruses. The present paper confirms this assumption and describes the isolation of an RSV which induces fusiform cell transformation and is free of overt avian leukosis viruses.

Materials and Methods. Virus. A stock of Bryan high-titer RSV containing Rous-associated virus type 3 [RSV (RAV-3)] was observed to produce a small fraction of foci with fusiform cell morphology. A purely fusiform line of RSV was derived from RSV(RAV-3) by several successive single-focus isolations. The fusiform stock was antigenically identical to RAV-3 and contained RAV-3 as an associated agent. From this stock a leukosis-free RSV was isolated as described below. It will be referred to as fRO, for fusiform RSV type O. The original type O RSV causes round cell transformation and will be abbreviated rRO. Neither fRO nor rRO belong to an established avian tumor virus subgroup (6, 7). Origin and production of the following viruses have been described previously: Rous-associated virus (RAV) types 1 and 5 (subgroup A), RAV-2 (subgroup B), RAV-7 (subgroup C), Carr–Zilber-associated virus (CZAV), and RAV-50 (subgroup D) (8, 9).

Cell cultures and virus assay. Source and susceptibility patterns of the avian cell types used have been described (9). The assay of RSV was carried out in the presence of 2 μg/ml polybrene (10).

Immunological techniques. Virus neutrali-

[1] Supported by U. S. Public Health Service Research Grant CA 10569 from the National Cancer Institute.

87

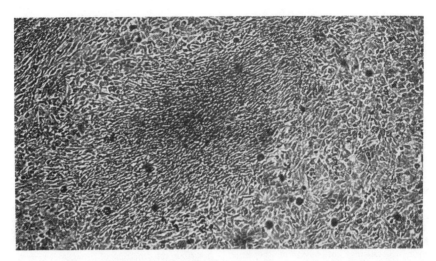

FIG. 1. Type C/A chick embryo fibroblast culture with a focus induced by fRO.

zation by antibody was determined by assaying for surviving focus formers after incubation at 37° for 40 min with appropriate serum dilutions. Fluorescent staining of infected cells was carried out without prior fixation. The details have been described (11, 12).

Results. Isolation of a leukosis-free Rous sarcoma virus causing fusiform cell transformation. Type C/B chick embryo fibroblasts were infected with a high dilution of fusiform RSV(RAV-3) yielding from 3–5 foci per 60-mm dish. The cultures were overlaid on the next day with nutrient agar containing a dilution of chicken serum sufficient to neutralize more than 99% of fusiform RSV(RAV-3). On day 7 foci were marked with a wax pencil, aspirated through the agar into the tip of a capillary pipette, and transferred onto normal C/B feeder cells. The plates containing isolated single foci were then transferred at 2- to 3-day intervals, and the growth medium was tested for the presence of free virus before each transfer. Of 110 foci tested 109 produced fusiform RSV of the parental serotype. One failed to release virus capable of transforming type C/O or C/B chick embryo fibroblasts but unlike the parental virus did produce foci on type C/A

cells. This host range is characteristic of rRO, and the observations described in this paper indicate that the new viral isolate is a mutant of rRO causing fusiform cell transformation. It will be referred to as fRO. The foci induced by fRO are illustrated in Fig. 1.

A stock preparation of fRO was grown in type C/A chick embryo fibroblasts and was tested for the presence of an avian leukosis virus by searching for an agent capable of interfering with focus formation by fRO (13). Two such tests failed to detect avian leukosis virus beyond the endpoint of transformation by fRO. This indicated that preparations of fRO did not contain a nontransforming avian tumor virus in amounts exceeding the titer of focus-forming virus. However, a low titered avian leukosis, preexisting in "normal" C/A cells could contribute to the envelope properties of fRO. This possibility is suggested by recent studies on rRO (15-16).

Host range of fRO. Among chicken cells only type C/A (line 7, Regional Poultry Laboratory, U.S.D.A., East Lansing, Michigan) was found regularly susceptible to fRO (Table I). However, titers of fRO in cultures derived from different individual C/A embryos varied. About two thirds of the em-

88

bryos yielded highly susceptible cultures. These were used as an arbitrary standard of susceptibility (relative efficiency of plating = 1). On one third of the C/A embryos titers of fRO were reduced from 5- to 20-fold. The same C/A embryos which were relatively resistant to fRO also showed a diminished susceptibility to rRO. High and reduced susceptibility of C/A cultures was a stable trait of the cells which persisted through several transfers.

C/O cultures could be divided into two categories: One was prevalent in a commercial line of White Leghorn embryos (Heisdorf and Nelson Farms, Redmond, Wash.) and was insusceptible to fRO. The other, represented by embryos of line 15I (Regional Poultry Laboratory, U.S.D.A., East Lansing, Mich.) showed a low but significant susceptibility to fRO. About 10% of the commercial C/O embryos also showed this low susceptibility. All C/O embryos, on which fRO induced foci, were also susceptible to rRO. Type C/B and C/AB chicken cells, known to be insusceptible to rRO were also uniformly resistant to fRO. Fibroblasts derived from Japanese quail or from ringneck pheasants were susceptible to fRO as they were to rRO. The host range of fRO is thus completely identical to that of rRO (6, 7, 14, 15).

Surface antigens of fRO. Several high-titered antisera produced in chickens against avian tumor virus subgroups A, B, C, and D failed to neutralize the infectivity of fRO. However, three sera prepared in ringneck pheasants against rRO also neutralized fRO. The titers of these sera against rRO and against fRO were identical. An antigenic relationship between fRO and rRO also was demonstrated by fluorescent antibody staining. All sera which specifically stained rRO-infected cells also reacted with fRO-infected cells.

Interference and facilitation. Table II summarizes the effects of avian leukosis viruses on the cellular susceptibility to fRO. Three types of responses were observed: (i) interference with fRO, (ii) unaltered cellular susceptibility, and (iii) facilitation of fRO infec-

TABLE I. Host Range of fRO.

Cell type	No. of embryos tested	Relative efficiency of plating[a]
Chicken		
C/A	12	0.05 to 1.0
C/O[b]	21	$<10^{-3}$
C/O[c]	7	1.3 to 8×10^{-2}
C/B	5	$<10^{-3}$
C/AB	3	$<10^{-3}$
Japanese quail	4	0.1 to 2.3
Ringneck pheasant	5	0.95 to 1.3

[a] The high plating efficiency found with most embryos of type C/A (Line 7, Regional Poultry Laboratory, U.S.D.A. East Lansing, Michigan) was arbitrarily set as 1.0.

[b] About 90% of the embryos from a White Leghorn line, Heisdorf and Nelson Farms, Redmond, Washington.

[c] All embryos of line 15I, Regional Poultry Laboratory, U.S.D.A. East Lansing, Michigan, and about 10% of the White Leghorn embryos, Heisdorf and Nelson Farms, Redmond, Washington.

tion. Interference with fRO was observed in C/A cultures preinfected with either subgroup B (RAV-2) or D (CZAV, RAV-50) avian leukosis viruses. This sensitivity to interference is identical to the one reported for rRO (7, 14). No significant change in cellular susceptibility to fRO was seen after preinfection of C/A cells with subgroup C leukosis viruses (RAV-7, RAV 49). Facilitation of infection with fRO was observed with C/O cells of line 15I. Whereas uninfected cultures of this type showed only a low susceptibility to fRO (Table I), preinfection of the cultures with subgroup A avian leukosis viruses brought the susceptibility up to the level of C/A cells (Table II). A similar facilitation on line 15I fibroblasts has been reported for rRO (18).

Ability of fRO to reproduce in solitary infection. The reproduction of infectious rRO has been reported to be influenced by the type of host cell which is infected. After infection with rRO some cell types release only noninfectious particles whereas others release infectious rRO (15, 16). The synthesis of fRO is similarly affected by the cell (Table III). Single foci produced by fRO in

89

TABLE II. Effects of Avian Leukosis Viruses on Cellular Susceptibility to fRO.[a]

Preinfecting avian leukosis virus	Cell type	Relative efficiency of plating
RAV-2	C/A	1×10^{-3}
CZAV	C/A	$<10^{-2}$
RAV-50	C/A	3×10^{-3}
RAV-7	C/A	1.2
RAV-1	C/O, line 15I	17
RAV-5	C/O, line 15I	30 to 55

[a] Chick embryo fibroblasts were infected with the avian leukosis viruses listed in the table, transferred three times at 2-day intervals and challenged with fRO. Efficiencies of plating are expressed in relation to uninfected control cultures of the same cell type. Successful infection with each of the leukosis viruses was verified by demonstrating interference with a Rous sarcoma virus of the respective subgroup.

Japanese quail fibroblast cultures were free of infectious virus. In contrast, most single foci isolated from type C/A chicken cells contained infectious fRO. This host dependence of reproduction seen with fRO and rRO will be considered more thoroughly in another report (17).

Production of pseudotypes with fRO. Chick embryo fibroblast cultures infected and transformed by fRO were superinfected with avian leukosis viruses of subgroups A, B, C, and D. The virus present in the culture fluids 4 days after superinfection was harvested and characterized with respect to host range, sensitivity to interference and reaction with subgroup-specific, neutralizing antibodies. The majority of the focus-forming virus in these harvests consisted of pseudotype particles whose envelope properties were controlled by the avian leukosis virus which had been used to superinfect the culture. Only a small percentage of focus formers (from 0.2–2%) had retained the host range of fRO. These observations demonstrate that fRO can undergo phenotypic mixing with avian leukosis viruses to yield pseudotype virions.

Oncogenicity of fRO in ringneck pheasants. In order to test whether a virus which produces fusiform foci in tissue culture can also induce sarcomas in the animal, about 5×10^{3} focus-forming units of fRO were injected into the wing web of 4-week-old ringneck pheasants. Three out of four animals developed sarcomas at the site of inoculation. Tissue sections were obtained from the tumors and stained with hematoxylin and eosin. A comparison with sections from sarcomas induced by rRO in the same species did not reveal conspicuous morphological differences of the tumor cells.

Discussion. Only one focus out of 110 was found to release fRO. The remainder produced fusiform RSV of the parental serotype. This was probably caused by the persistence of RAV in the majority of the foci picked, but further studies are necessary to confirm this assumption. Although no overt helper virus was detectable in stocks of fRO, the synthesis of infectious fRO progeny may nevertheless depend on some auxiliary genetic material which could preexist in the cell. The finding that infectious fRO is released from C/A but not from Japanese quail cells is in accordance with this suggestion. A similar dependence of reproduction on cell type has been found for rRO by Weiss (14) and by Hanafusa and co-workers (16). Weiss also observed that the cells capable of synthesizing infectious rRO contained the avian tumor virus group-specific antigen prior to infection. This antigen may indicate the presence of viral genetic material in the cells, although a complete virus has not been detected so far.

TABLE III. Virus Production in Foci Induced by fRO.[a]

Cell type	Number of embryos tested	Fraction of single foci-producing fRO
C/A	3	25/30
Japanese quail	7	0/48

[a] Chick or quail embryo fibroblast cultures were infected with a high dilution of fRO giving 10 foci or less per 35-mm petri dish. At day 7 foci were picked, and transferred singly into test tubes. The cells were destroyed by sonication and the presence of cell-free infectious virus in the focus was demonstrated by assay on quail fibroblasts.

The envelope-controlled properties of fRO and rRO were found to be identical. This plus the fact that both agents were derived from the Bryan high-titer strain of RSV makes it likely that they represent mutants of the same virus, differing in the gene which controls the shape of the transformed cell. Since fusiform and round foci produced in the same culture are easily distinguishable, the two mutants differing in this marker should prove useful in future genetic experiments.

Summary. A Rous sarcoma virus (RSV) is described which shares the envelope properties of RSV type O but causes infected cells to assume a fusiform shape. The agent induces sarcomas in susceptible birds. Japanese quail cells infected with a single particle of this virus fail to yield infectious progeny whereas chicken cells of type C/A readily reproduce the agent.

The authors thank Mr. R. Raymond of Heisdorf and Nelson Farms for his generous help in obtaining chicken embryos of known genetic constitution. Japanese quail eggs were kindly provided by Dr. W. M. Farrow of Life Sciences, Inc., St. Petersburg, Florida. Mrs. Susan Norwood and Mrs. Sally Olson rendered competent technical assistance.

1. Temin, H. M., Virology 10, 182 (1960).

2. Temin, H. M., Virology 13, 158 (1961).

3. Purchase, H. G., and Okazaki, W., J. Nat. Cancer Inst. 32, 579 (1964).

4. Vogt, P. K., *in* "Perspectives in Virology" (M. Pollard, ed.), Vol. 5, p. 199. Harper & Row, New York (1967).

5. Hanafusa, H., Hanafusa, T., and Rubin, H., Proc. Nat. Acad. Sci. U.S.A. 51, 41 (1964).

6. Weiss, R. A., Virology 32, 719 (1967).

7. Vogt, P. K., Proc. Nat. Acad. Sci. U.S.A. 58, 801 (1967).

8. Ishizaki, R., and Vogt, P. K., Virology 30, 375 (1966).

9. Duff, R. G., and Vogt, P. K., Virology 39, 18 (1969).

10. Toyoshima, K., and Vogt, P. K., Virology 38, 414 (1969).

11. Kelloff, G., and Vogt, P. K., Virology 29, 377 (1966).

12. Vogt, P. K., *in* "Fundamental Techniques in Virology" (K. Habel and N. P. Salzman, eds.), p. 316. Academic Press, New York (1969).

13. Rubin, H., and Vogt, P. K., Virology 17, 184 (1962).

14. Weiss, R. A., J. Gen. Virol. 5, 511 (1969).

15. Weiss, R. A., J. Gen. Virol. 5, 529 (1969).

16. Hanafusa, T., Miyamoto, T., and Hanafusa, H., Virology 40, 55 (1970).

17. Vogt, P. K., and Friis, R. R., Virology, in press. (1970).

18. Ishizaki, R., and Shimizu, T., Virology 40, 415 (1970).

Radio-Induced Mutants of the Schmidt-Ruppin Strain of Rous Sarcoma Virus

ALICE GOLDÉ

INTRODUCTION

Previous experiments performed with a nonclonal Schmidt-Ruppin strain of Rous sarcoma virus (SR-RSV) (Goldé and Latarjet, 1966) have shown that the oncogenic and virus producing capacities coded by the viral genome can be dissociated by irradiation with high doses of γ-rays. Indeed, nonproducing (NP) transformed cells were obtained after infection of chick embryo fibroblasts by several irradiated suspensions of SR-RSV, suggesting that some surviving virions were still able to transform cells but unable to give rise to progeny. Furthermore, NP cells never released any virions even after superinfection with avian leukosis viruses. Therefore, it was suggested that oncogenic and virus-producing capacities of RSV can be expressed and replicated independently

The experiments to be presented here were performed with clonal SR-RSV, and their first purpose was to confirm earlier findings, particularly the production of transformed NP cells, and to complete them by showing that these NP cells were really cancerous cells. A second purpose was to isolate a mutant still able to replicate, but which would have lost transforming and oncogenic capacities, in agreement with the hypothesis of the independence of both functions previously raised.

As will be seen, NP cells were obtained again, and it is shown that several NP cell strains were able to produce graft tumors on the CAM of embryonated eggs; on the other hand, a nononcogenic mutant, called nontransforming γ [NT (γ)] virus was isolated from the heavily irradiated suspensions, and its characteristics suggest that it is the parental SR-RSV having lost the oncogenic capacity after γ-rays.

MATERIALS AND METHODS

Viruses. All clonal strains of SR-RSV were isolated from a nonclonal strain kindly supplied by Dr. J. R. C. Harris, and belonging to the subgroup D of the avian oncogenic viruses, as shown by Duff and Vogt (1969).

All the other strains of standard virus,

except B-RSV (RAV 1), were clonal strains kindly supplied by Dr. H Hanafusa.

The following abbreviations will be used: SR-RSV = Schmidt-Ruppin strain Rous sarcoma virus; B-RSV = Bryan strain Rous sarcoma virus; RAV = Rous associated virus; B-RSV (RAV 1) and B-RSV (RAV 2) = pseudotypes of B-RSV coated with a RAV 1 or RAV 2 envelope.

γ-Rays. A colbat-60 source delivering 7500 r per minute in the irradiated sample was used. All irradiations were performed under conditions of inactivation by direct effect. These conditions are fulfilled when RSV is dispersed in a medium containing 10% calf serum and frozen at −76° at the time of irradiation by immersion in a carbo-ice-alcohol mixture. After irradiation, the viral suspension was thawed, diluted with M 199 plus 10% calf serum, incubated 15 min at 37° and inoculated immediately

Cell cultures. Chick embryo cell cultures were prepared as described by Rubin (1960), from individual Brown Leghorn embryos, lymphomatosis free and genetically susceptible to the A, B, C, and D subgroups of avian tumor viruses (C/O type) (Vogt and Ishizaki, 1965; Duff and Vogt, 1969).

The standard medium was composed of 10% calf serum, 5% calf embryo extract, and 85% M 199. For subcultures and infection of the suspensions of trypsinized cells, the medium was composed of 10% tryptose phosphate broth, 5% calf serum and 85% M 199.

Virus assays. The virus content of culture media was measured by two methods. (1) Inoculation on the chorioallantoic membrane of lymphomatosis-free chick embryos. Pocks produced after 7 days were counted (Rubin, 1955), titers being expressed as pock-forming units (PFU) per milliliter. (2) Infection of chick embryo cells, 0.2–1.0 ml of inoculum being added to 1.2 × 10⁶ trypsinized cells suspended in 5 ml of medium. and seeded in a 60-mm petri dish. The infected cultures were overlaid with 6 ml of agar medium 18–24 hours after infection, and foci of transformed cells were counted after 6 and 7 days (Temin and Rubin, 1958) Results are expressed in focus-forming units (FFU) per milliliter.

Virus-producing cells, or infective centers (IC) were assayed *in vitro* (Rubin, 1960) as follows: First, the infected cell monolayer was rinsed about 5 hours with fresh nutritive medium, to elute the adsorbed virus; then, the cells were trypsinized, counted, and irradiated with a dose of γ-rays of 5000 r. A known number of irradiated cells was seeded with 1.2 × 10⁶ trypsinized fibroblasts, and the cultures were overlaid with agar as for the virus assay. Results are expressed as the number of virus-producing cells per 100 irradiated cells. The virus production of each infective center was calculated from the number of virus-producing cells per culture and the titer of free virus released in the medium 20 hours before assay.

Cloning method. Clonal and subclonal virus strains were obtained either from cultured pocks (Goldé, 1965) or from foci of transformed cells produced by irradiated surviving virions. Foci were harvested from dishes containing no more than 5 foci. A hole was made in agar above the colony, and transformed cells were harvested with diluted trypsin and seeded with 10⁶ uninfected cells per dish by the standard method.

RESULTS

Alteration of the Virus-Producing Capacity after γ-Rays

The action of different doses of γ-rays on the virus producing capacity of clonal and subclonal SR-RSV was estimated from the virus yield of cultures of single pocks or foci induced by surviving virions.

The study of the pock cultures showed that the percentage of nonproducing pocks increased with the dose of γ-rays (Table 1). Nonproducer foci of Rous cells (about 20%) were also obtained in chick embryo fibroblast cultures infected with SR-RSV irradiated at 3000 kr, but the dose effect of γ-rays was not studied as in the case of pocks. Among focus cultures that remained virus producers, the smaller virus yield was observed at the higher doses of γ-rays (Table 2). These results are in close agreement with those previously obtained by irradiating nonclonal SR-RSV (Goldé and Latarjet, 1966). Furthermore, there was a variable

TABLE 1

PERCENTAGE OF NONPRODUCING POCKS AS A
FUNCTION OF γ-RAYS DOSE ON A CLONAL
STRAIN OF SR-RSV $(S_4)^a$

γ-Rays dose (kr)	Survival of PFU (%)	Number of pocks studied	Nonproducing pocks (%)
900	10	11	0
2000	2.5	8	12.5
3000	0.1	8	25

[a] The culture medium of cells infected with
SR-RSV clonal strain S_4 was irradiated at various
doses. The irradiated viral suspension was then
inoculated on the CAM. Pocks produced after 7
days were counted and cultivated individually
with noninfected-chick embryo fibroblasts. The
culture media were assayed in totality 2 weeks
later.

TABLE 2

VIRUS YIELD OF CHICK EMBRYO FIBROBLASTS
INFECTED WITH SUBCLONAL STRAINS OBTAINED
AFTER IRRADIATION OF CLONAL STRAIN OF
SR-RSV[a]

Parental clone of SR-RSV	Virus yield (control) before γ-Rays	γ-ray doses (kr)	Relative virus yield of cells infected by subclonal strains of irradiated or nonirradiated virus[b] (2)
TB₂	1	0	0.07 0.25 0.25 0.5 0.5 0.8 1
S₄	1	900	0.025 0.05 0.2 0.25 0.25
		3000	0.02 0.02 0.02 0.04
S₁Cl₃	1	3000	0.0005 0.0007 0.0007 0.003 0.001 0.012 0.015 0.05 0.1

[a] Foci of transformed cells, produced either by
a nonirradiated clonal strain (TB₂) or by irradiated clonal strains of SR-RSV (S₁Cl₃ and S₄) were
isolated and cultivated during 2 weeks with chick
embryo fibroblasts. The virus content of the
medium was subsequently measured by CAM
assay, and compared with that of cultures infected with the nonirradiated parental virus (control). The titers of controls were 5000 (TB₂), 2000
(S₄), and 4000 (S₁Cl₃) FFU per 10^5 cells.
[b] Each figure is the relative production of a
different subclone and the mean of two replicate
cultures.

decrease of the yield among cultures infected
with different clonal virus strains isolated
from the same irradiated parental virus
(Table 2). This was presumably not a

radiation effect since a similar heterogeneity
could be observed among cultures infected
with 7 subclonal nonirradiated virus strains
(TB₂, Table 2), an observation agreeing
with that of Vogt (1967) on B-RSV (0)

*Tumorigenicity of NP Cells Produced by
Defective Transforming Virions*

The NP cells obtained by inoculating
irradiated viral suspensions either on the
CAM or on chicken cells *in vitro* were small
round cells multiplying on top of the associated embryo fibroblasts with which they
were maintained and weekly subcultured,
except for one strain, which was composed
of large epithelioid cells (Cl₂d, Table 3). As
mentioned previously (Goldé and Latarjet,
1966) any NP cell strain released virus after
superinfection with saturating doses of RAV1
or RAV50, when checked *in vitro* by inoculating the culture medium in totality each
day during the following 4 days, before
claiming that these cells were really
cancerous cells, it was necessary to check
their tumorigenicity. For this purpose, the
chorioallantoic membrane was chosen rather
than chicken since Temin (1962) showed that
NP cells issued from the B-RSV strain gave
tumors as well on the CAM as in chicken, and
to avoid an eventual elimination of cells
related with nonhistocompatibility. Therefore, the tumorigenicity of six clonal NP cell
strains was tested by their ability to give
graft tumors on the CAM of 10-day-old
chick embryos and measured by the number
of cells giving one graft tumor (tumorigenic
dose). Results, reported in Table 3, show
that tumorigenic doses were comparable for
the various cell strains except for the pock
culture No. 26. In fact, the true tumorigenic
doses were at least 3 times smaller than those
reported in the table, since transformed cells
were associated with noninfected fibroblasts
in the proportion of about 1 to 2. In parallel
controls, the inoculation of 1×10^6/CAM
noninfected chick embryo fibroblasts never
gave any tumor. Some tumors, harvested
and cultivated, gave again small transformed cells with the same appearance and
tumorigenicity as the parental pock cells
(Table 3, No. 10).

94

TABLE 3

TUMORIGENICITY OF NONPRODUCING CHICKEN CELLS TRANSFORMED BY ONCOGENIC
NONPRODUCTIVE VIRIONS OBTAINED FROM IRRADIATED SR-RSV[a]

Parental virus strain	γ-Ray doses (kr)	Origin of the transformed cells	Time of culture before inoculation on CAM (days)	Cell number/CAM number	Total number of tumors	Tumorigenic doses[b]
Nonclonal SR-RSV	2100	Pock (A2)	45	$1.8 \times 10^6/4$	3	600,000
		Pock (10)	35	$5 \times 10^5/3$	2	250,000
		Tumor (10)	10	$1.8 \times 10^5/3$	1	180,000
		Pock (11)	35	$5 \times 10^5/3$	3	170,000
		Pock (21)	35	$4.8 \times 10^5/3$	3	160,000
		Pock (21)	50	$2.5 \times 10^6/7$	17	150,000
Clonal SR-RSV (TB$_2$)	2000	Focus (Cl$_2$d)	37	$1.6 \times 10^6/8$	13	120,000
Clonal SR-RSV (S$_1$Cl$_3$)	3000	Pock (26)	28	$1.2 \times 10^7/6$	6	2×10^6

[a] Nonproducing pocks or foci of NP transformed cells were obtained by infection of CAM or chick embryo fibroblasts with irradiated viral suspensions of clonal or nonclonal SR-RSV strains. These pocks and foci were cultivated and transferred periodically at the same time as noninfected cells. A definite number of transformed cells were inoculated on the CAM after a culture time of 10–50 days, and 8 days later, the graft-tumors were counted and explanted *in vitro*.

[b] Tumorigenic dose = mean number of cells required to give one graft-tumor on the CAM. In fact, the tumorigenic doses are about 3 times lower than those reported here, since transformed, nonproducing cells constituted no more than a third of the inoculated cell population (see text).

Study of the Low-Titer Virus Subclones

As seen in the first part of this paper, the low titer mutants were isolated from viral suspensions irradiated with the higher doses of γ-rays (Table 2), that is, suspensions containing sterile oncogenic virions too. Therefore, the hypothesis was raised that the low-titer mutants had genomes partially defective for the capacity to replicate, the number of radio-induced lesions increasing with the dose and knocking out an increasing number of informations until virions were deprived of reproductive capacity. In this case, one could expect that cultures infected by low-titer viruses would contain a number of infective centers comparable to that of cultures infected by the parental nonirradiated virus, but with a much lower virus yield per center. In order to check this hypothesis and this prediction, the number of infective centers and the virus production were studied in cultures infected with low-titer mutants as follows:

Before irradiating and subcloning a clonal SR-RSV strain, it was checked that three clonal SR-RSV strains were specifically neutralized by SR-RSV antiserum (Table 4), and therefore belonged to the same

TABLE 4

ANTIBODY NEUTRALIZATION OF CLONAL
STRAINS OF SR-RSV[a]

Virus strain	Serum					
	Anti RAV 1		Anti RAV 2		Anti SR-RSV	
	Dilution	Survival	Dilution	Survival	Dilution	Survival
Homologous virus[b]	1:1000	0.0003	1:1000	0.01	1:100	0.01
S$_1$Cl$_3$[c]	1:1000	1	1:1000	1	1:100	0.06
S$_1$Cl$_4$	1:1000	0.6	1:1000	0.6	1:100	0.06
S$_1$Cl$_6$	1:1000	1	1:1000	0.7	1:100	0.06

[a] A 1:100 or 1:1000 dilution of serum was incubated at 37° for 40 min with about 5×10^5 PFU of each virus strain, then assayed on the CAM. Results are expressed as the fraction of virus surviving.

[b] (B-RSV (RAV 1), B-RSV (RAV 2), SR-RSV).

[c] Data are the mean of two separate experiments.

antigenic subgroup D as the nonclonal parental strain. One clonal strain was then chosen randomly (S$_1$Cl$_3$), irradiated at 3000 kr, and a first cloning was performed after

TABLE 5

PEDIGREE OF THE DIFFERENT SUBCLONAL IRRADIATED VIRUS STRAINS STUDIED IN TABLES 6 AND 7

S_1Cl_3 γ-rays, 3000 kr			subclonal strain from one focus
C_5 (normal titer)	C_{17} (low titer)	C_{18} (low titer)	1st cloning (foci) after γ-rays
2-5	3-4-7-14	2-3-8	2nd cloning (foci)

irradiation to detect normal titer and low-titer virus subclones among several cultures of transformed foci. A second cloning was then performed from one normal titer and two low-titer virus subclones (Table 5). Foci harvested at the second cloning were mixed with noninfected chick embryo fibroblasts, and the virus yield and infective centers were assayed 18 days later. Normal chick embryo fibroblasts were periodically added, particularly when the mixed cultures were subcultured, to promote infection and transformation. Results are recorded in Table 6.

One can see that the normal-titer clone (C_5) gave normal-titer subclones, whereas low-titer clones (C_{17} and C_{18}) gave low-titer subclones; furthermore, the order of magnitude of the virus production of the latter depended closely on that of cultures infected with virus from the parental clone.

On the other hand, the virus yield depended on both the number of infective centers and the virus production per infective center. Thus, several cultures infected with low-titer virus contained a much lower percentage of infective centers than cultures infected with the C_5 normal titer clone or the S_1Cl_3 nonirradiated parental clone; however, several transfers had been performed to enhance the spreading of virus to surrounding cells. Therefore, the question was raised: Was an inhibiting substance or were interfering particles released in the culture medium which prevented the reinfection? This latter hypothesis was tested in the following experiments.

Interfering, Infectious Viral Particles Isolated from the Nutritive Medium of Low-Titer Virus-Infected Cultures

The media of cultures infected with three low-titer and one normal-titer virus subclones were tested for the presence of inter-fering particles, controls being the media of S_1Cl_3-parental virus cultures and of noninfected chick embryo fibroblasts. The procedure used was that described by Rubin and Vogt (1962) for the *in vitro* assay of avian leukosis viruses.

Separate groups of chick embryo fibroblasts, issued from a single chick embryo, were infected in suspension with the infectious culture media, diluted so as to have less than one FFU per petri dish. One of them remained uninfected and served as a standard of host sensitivity. After 7 days, and two transfers, each set of cultures was superinfected in suspension with standard RSV belonging to subgroups A, B, and D. Agar medium was added 20 hours later, and foci were counted after 7 days.

Table 7 contains the results from representative experiments. One can see that the plating efficiencies of the challenge viruses belonging to both B [RSV (RAV2)] and D [SR-RSV] subgroups were much lower in plates preinfected with diluted medium of cultures of each of the three low-titer mutants in which no foci appeared, than in plates preinfected with the medium of the normal titer mutant or of the nonirradiated parental virus cultures. These results show that 1 ml of the 10^{-6} diluted medium of each of the low-titer virus-infected cultures contained at least one infectious unit of an interfering virus which replicated before addition of the challenge virus and induced cellular resistance against two antigenic types of RSV. This virus was called NT (nontransforming) γ virus.

Furthermore, one could observe a slight reduction, at the lowest dilution of the preinfecting virus, of the plating efficiency of RSV belonging to the A subgroup [B-RAV1)] in the low-titer-virus preinfected sets.

Chick embryo fibroblasts infected solely

TABLE 6

Growth in C/O Chick Embryo Fibroblasts of Subclonal Virus Strains Obtained after Irradiation at 3000 kr of the S_1Cl_3 Clonal Strain

Virus strains (clones or subclones)	Number of subcultures before assays	Virus production (FFU/10^5 cells)	IC (%)	FFU/IC
$S_1Cl_3{}^a$ (A)	0	6×10^3	59	0.11
(B)	0	6×10^3	21	0.3
$C_5{}^b$	2	3×10^3	ND^c	—
C_{5-2}	3	1.6×10^4	90	0.18
C_{5-5}	1	1.3×10^4	45	0.2
C_{17}	2	2×10^1	ND	—
C_{17-3}	2	2.4×10^2	4	0.06
C_{17-4}	2	7×10^2	20	0.035
C_{17-7}	1	0.55×10^2	1	0.05
C_{17-14}	2	0.5×10^1	0.1	0.001
C_{18}	2	2.5×10^2	ND	—
C_{18-2}	0	1.4×10^3	15	0.1
C_{18-3}	0	7×10^2	14	0.55
C_{18-8}	0	4×10^2	5	0.075

^{a} S_1Cl_3 is the parental clonal virus strains. (A) and (B) are two separate experiments in which multiplicities of infection were respectively 0.05 and 0.005 FFU/cell. Assays were performed 7 days after infection.

^{b} C_5, C_{17}, and C_{18} are virus subclones isolated from S_1Cl_3 irradiated at 3000 kr; each of them has been recloned to give subclonal strains. Free virus and infective centers (IC) were assayed 18 days after infection of chick embryo fibroblasts with each subclonal virus strain. Data are the mean of two separate experiments.

^{c} ND, not done.

with NT (γ) virus had a normal appearance and gave no graft tumor on the CAM. They contained the group-specific (GS) antigen of avian tumor viruses, as titrated by the COFAL test (Sarma e al., 1964), in amount comparable with that detected in the same number of RAV1-infected cells used as controls.

On the other hand, preinfection of cells with the diluted medium of C_5 infected-cells enhanced slightly the plating efficiency of each challenge virus: the meaning of this observation is under investigation

DISCUSSION

That infection of chick embryo fibroblasts with irradiated clonal SR-RSV results in the appearance of nonproducing transformed cells agrees with previous results obtained with irradiated nonclonal SR-RSV (Goldé and Latarjet, 1966). The fact that these NP cells gave graft tumors shows that they were truly neoplastic cells, produced by infection with radiation-induced nonproductive oncogenic virions, the defectiveness of which presumably resulted from the destruction or alteration of the part of the viral genome coding for the virus-producing capacity. Moreover, the failure to induce the production of virions by superinfecting NP cells with avian leukosis viruses suggests that the defectiveness of the defective genome, eventually persisting in the cell, is not compen-

TABLE 7

Relative Plating Efficiencies of A, B, and D Antigenic Types of RSV on Chicken Cells Preinfected with Diluted Culture Medium of Parental and Radio-Induced Virus-Infected Cells^a

Preinfecting subclonal virus strains	Culture medium		Relative plating efficiencies		
	FFU/ml	Dilution factor	B-RSV (RAV1)	B-RSV (RAV2)	SR-RSV (S_1Cl_3)
None	—	—	1	1	1
S_1Cl_3	9×10^4	10^{-6}	1	1	0.7
		10^{-7}	1	1	1
C_{5-2}	2×10^5	10^{-7}	1.2	2.6	1.8
C_{17-3}	3.5×10^3	10^{-5}	0.3	<0.01	<0.006
		10^{-6}	1	<0.05	<0.02
C_{17-14}	10^1	10^{-2}	0.25	<0.07	<0.01
		10^{-5}	1	<0.05	<0.02
		10^{-6}	1	<0.05	<0.02
C_{18-8}	5×10^3	10^{-5}	0.25	<0.01	<0.006
		10^{-6}	1	<0.05	<0.02

^{a} Plating efficiencies in control cells not preinfected with diluted infectious medium = 1.0, the mean number of foci per plate being 155, B-RSV (RAV1); 90, B-RSV (RAV2); and 151 (SR-RSV). The culture medium of cells infected with the parental nonirradiated S_1Cl_3 strain and subclonal viral strains obtained after irradiation of S_1Cl_3 at 3000 kr, were assayed and diluted to contain less than 1 FFU/ml. Then 0.5 ml of each diluted medium was added to infect 1.5×10^6 chick embryo fibroblasts, which were challenged 7 days later, after two transfers, with RSV belonging to A, B, or D antigenic types, under the conditions described for the focus assay. Data are the mean of replicate cultures.

sated by phenotypic mixing as observed with RSV (0) (Vogt, 1967).

Concerning the hypothesis of the partial defectiveness of the genome of the low-titer mutants, raised when these experiments were undertaken, it is neither confirmed nor excluded by present results. One has seen that the low titer found at the population level may be explained by the presence of the interfering NT (γ) virus which, by preventing the spread of the SR-RSV progeny through the cell population, prevents also the increase of the number of infective centers. However, the low yield per infective center in some mutants (Table 6) could be due either to an interference phenomenon between SR-RSV and γ virions, the latter having a much higher titer than the former, or to a partial defectiveness of the SR-RSV genome.

What is the possible origin of the NT (γ) virus?

First, it is a virus belonging to the group of avian oncogenic viruses; indeed, preliminary studies show that it is specifically neutralized by antisera against B and D subgroups; it has the same morphology and contains a heavy RNA with a sedimentation coefficient of 65–70 S (unpublished results from Dr Montagnier) as other RSV. Furthermore, it was seen that cells where NT (γ) virus replicates solely contain "gs" antigen. There remains the hypothesis that NT (γ) virus could be a contaminating lymphomatosis virus. It has been seen that it induces a high resistance against B and D subgroup of RSV, D subgroup being the subgroup to which the parental SR-RSV belongs. Since an interference can take place between subgroups B and D (Duff and Vogt, 1969), the NT (γ) virus behaves as a lymphomatosis virus belonging to subgroup D (like RAV 50). However, our attempts to isolate a RAV 50 from the parental SR-RSV by the end-point dilution method always failed (see Table 7), which is a strong argument against the hypothesis of a contaminating RAV 50. On the other hand, the contamination with RAV 50 after harvesting of the low-titer mutants can be excluded, since this lymphomatosis virus was not being studied in the laboratory when these experiments were performed.

Concerning the slight resistance induced by NT (γ) virus against subgroup A of RSV, recent results of neutralization experiments suggest that it is related to the presence of some virions belonging to the subgroup A, and not with a cytopathic effect produced by the replicating NT (γ) virus. Although improbable, the hypothesis of a contamination with RAV 1 cannot be excluded. Other experiments are necessary to check this point.

Therefore, the most likely explanation remains that NT (γ) virus belongs to subgroup D and is the parental SR-RSV in which γ-rays have knocked out the oncogenic capacity. In addition, γ-rays may have inactivated an information for the synthesis of a repressor of the viral multiplication, since the titer of NT (γ) virus, measured in interfering units against subgroups D and B of RSV, is at least 100 times higher than that of the parental SR-RSV, expressed in FFU, for a same number of cells.

Present results, by showing the ability to obtain by γ-rays two classes of mutants, one lacking oncogenicity and the other virus-producing capacity, suggest that these two functions are coded by parts of the viral genome which can be replicated and translated independently. They further raise the problem whether the viral RNA molecule is composed of independent subunits. Recent biochemical studies have shown that the viral RNA of RSV, the molecular weight of which is 10^7 daltons (Robinson et al., 1967) can be broken in pieces of about 2.5×10^6 daltons (Duesberg, 1968; Montagnier et al., 1969). On the other hand, the X-ray inactivation curve of the oncogenic capacity of RSV (Latarjet and Chamaillard, 1962) had allowed to calculate that the size of the corresponding RNA target should be about 2.5×10^6 daltons too (Latarjet and Chamaillard, 1962). The close agreement between these results obtained with two different methods supports the hypothesis that the oncogenic capacity could be coded by one subunit representing one-fourth of the RNA molecule. Moreover, the fact that both mutants were isolated from the same heavily irradiated viral suspension suggests that the respective radiosensitivities of both involved functions are comparable. Therefore, the virus-producing capacity, like the oncogenic capacity, could be coded by an independent subunit one-fourth the size of the whole RNA molecule. This hypothesis is speculative, but experimentally testable.

ACKNOWLEDGMENTS

I wish to express my gratitude to Dr. Bataillon, who performed the COFAL tests; to Miss Jacqueline Villaudy and Miss Jeanine Crochet for their competent technical assistance.

This work was carried out with the financial support of the INSERM and of the Commissariat á l'Energie Atomique.

REFERENCES

DUESBERG, P. (1968). Physical properties of Rous sarcoma virus RNA. *Proc. Natl. Acad. Sci. U.S.* **60**, 1511–1518.

DUFF, R. G., and VOGT, P. K. (1969). Characteristics of two new avian tumor virus sub-groups. *Virology* **39**, 18–30.

GOLDÉ, A. (1965). Mise en évidence de la défectivité du virus de Rous par des cultures de pocks. *Compt. Rend. Acad. Sci. Paris* **262D**, 3507–3510.

GOLDÉ, A., and LATARJET, R. (1966). Dissociation, par irradiation, des fonctions oncogène et infectieuse du virus de Rous, souche de Schmidt-Ruppin. *Compt. Rend. Acad. Sci. Paris* **262D**, 420–424.

LATARJET, R., and CHAMAILLARD, L. (1962). Inactivation du virus de Friend par les rayons X et les ultra-violets. *Bull. Cancer* **49**, 382–389.

MONTAGNIER, L., GOLDÉ, A., and VIGIER, P. (1969). A possible subunit structure of Rous sarcoma virus RNA. *J. Gen. Virol.* **4**, 244–252.

ROBINSON, W. S., ROBINSON, H. L., and DUESBERG, P. (1967). Tumor virus RNA's. *Proc. Natl. Acad. Sci. U.S.* **58**, 825–834.

RUBIN, H. (1955). Quantitative relations between causative virus and cells in the Rous n° 1 chicken sarcoma. *Virology* **1**, 445–473.

RUBIN, H. (1960). An analysis of the assay of Rous sarcoma cells in vitro by the infectious center technique. *Virology* **10**, 29–49.

RUBIN, H., and VOGT, P. K. (1962). An avian leukosis virus associated with stocks of Rous sarcoma virus. *Virology* **17**, 184–194.

SARMA, P. S., HUEBNER, R. J., and ARMSTRONG, D. (1964). A simplified tissue culture tube neutralization test for Rous sarcoma virus antibodies. *Proc. Exptl. Soc. Biol. Med.* **115**, 481–486.

TEMIN, H. M. (1962). Separation of morphological conversion and virus production in Rous sarcoma virus infection. *Cold Spring Harbor Symp. Quant. Biol.* **27**, 407–414.

TEMIN, H. M., and RUBIN, H. (1958). Characteristics of an assay for Rous sarcoma virus and Rous sarcoma cells in tissue culture. *Virology* **6**, 669–688.

VOGT, P. K. (1967). A virus released by "nonproducing" Rous sarcoma cells. *Proc. Natl. Acad. Sci. U.S.* **58**, 801–808.

VOGT, P. K., and ISHIZAKI, R. (1965). Reciprocal patterns of genetic resistance to avian tumor viruses in two lines of chickens. *Virology* **26**, 664–672.

PROTEIN COMPONENTS

Glycoprotein Components of Avian and Murine RNA Tumor Viruses[1]

PETER H. DUESBERG, G. STEVEN MARTIN AND PETER K. VOGT

INTRODUCTION

Chemical analysis of purified avian myeloblastosis virus, a member of the avian tumor virus group, has indicated that there are 1.9 moles of glucosamine per 100 moles of total amino acids in the virus particle (Bonar and Beard, 1959; Purcell et al., 1962; Baluda and Nayak, 1969). The functional or structural viral component with which the carbohydrate is associated has not been determined. A recent analysis of the proteins obtained from several avian tumor viruses has shown the occurrence of two major and

several minor electrophoretically separable protein components in the virus. The two major components were found to react with antibody against the group-specific antigen of the avian tumor viruses (Duesberg et al., 1968). A specific protein or protein derivative which might represent the outer, type-specific viral antigen involved in virus neutralization by antibody (Ishizaki and Vogt, 1966; Vogt, 1970) was not reported. However, recently Tozawa et al. (1970) have shown that Tween 20-disrupted preparations of virus contain a trypsin-sensitive component, which specifically inhibits neutralizing antibody to the virus.

The present investigation describes two glycoproteins associated with purified preparations of avian and murine RNA tumor viruses. These glycoproteins are either sub-

[1] This investigation was supported by U.S. Public Health Service research grants CA 11426, CA 05619, and CA 10569 from the National Cancer Institute, and by a grant from the Jane Coffin Childs Memorial Fund for Medical Research.

group- or type-specific. The glycoproteins derived from members of different avian tumor virus subgroups can be distinguished by their electrophoretic properties. Viral glycoprotein-containing fractions with sedimentation coefficients of about 8 S and 4–2 S were found to inhibit virus neutralization by antibody.

MATERIALS AND METHODS

Viruses and cells. The Bryan high-titer strain of RSV was described previously (Duesberg *et al.*, 1968). It consists predominantly of RAV-1 and RSV(RAV-1), which belong to the subgroup A of avian tumor viruses (Ishizaki and Vogt, 1966; Vogt, 1970). It was abbreviated B-RSV(RAV-1). The Schmidt-Ruppin strain of RSV was also a member of avian tumor virus subgroup A and was abbreviated SR-RSV-A. The Prague-RSV is a member of subgroup C (Duff and Vogt, 1969; Vogt, 1970) and was abbreviated PR-RSV-C. The leukosis virus-free RSV derived from the Bryan strain was referred to as RSV(O) (Vogt, 1967a). Stocks of this virus were grown in type C/A chick embryo fibroblasts (Vogt and Ishizaki, 1965).

The B-RSV(RAV-1), SR-RSV-A, and PR-RSV-C were all grown on C/B or C/O (Vogt and Ishizaki, 1965; Vogt, 1970) cells of chicken embryos obtained from Kimber Farms (Fremont, California). All RSV-producing chick fibroblast cultures were started with 5–10 × 10^5 cells per 10-cm plastic petri dish in 10 ml of medium 199 supplemented with 2% tryptose-phosphate broth, 1% calf serum, 1% chicken serum (heated for 1 hour at 56°), and 0.5 µg of fungizone per milliliter (Grand Island Biological) (Rubin, 1960). The cells were infected with 0.5–1 ml stock virus at the time of seeding or several hours afterward. Stock virus was the medium of completely transformed cultures. Beginning 2 days after infection the medium was changed daily. Two to 3 days after infection, when between 30% (SR-RSV-A) and 80% (B-RSV(RAV-1)) of the cells were transformed, medium 199 containing 10% tryptose-phosphate broth and either 5% calf serum or 4% calf serum and 1% chick serum was used. For the propagation of PR-RSV-C the medium contained 2 µg/ml polybrene

(Abbott Laboratories, North Chicago, Illinois) (Toyoshima and Vogt, 1969), and the medium containing high concentration of serum was only used after >90% of the cells were transformed to minimize detachment of partially transformed cultures from the culture dish.

The Rauscher mouse leukemia virus (MLV) was propagated in the infected JLS-V5 or JLS-V9 cell line (kindly provided by Dr. F. Rauscher, National Cancer Institute) as described previously (Duesberg and Robinson, 1966) except for a change in the medium. The medium was Dulbecco's modified MEM (Grand Island Biological Company) containing 15% calf serum and 50 units of mycostatin per milliliter (Grand Island Biological Company).

Rous virus assay. The Rous sarcoma viruses were assayed as described previously (Rubin, 1960) except that when SR-RSV-A was assayed the agar overlay was supplemented with 3 mg/ml glucose, and an extra 4 ml of agar overlay was added after 4 days' incubation.

Antibody against SR-RSV-A was prepared by injecting 6-week-old chickens with approximately 1000 focus-forming units of SR-RSV-A. Birds in which the tumors regressed were bled for antiserum. Dilutions were made in medium 199 containing 2% tryptose-phosphate broth and 1% calf serum (199-2-1).

Inhibition of neutralizing antibody by materials released from disrupted virus. Fractions from sucrose gradients were pooled and dialyzed 1–2 days against Tris-saline (contains per liter, NaCl 8 g, KCl 0.38 g, Na$_2$HPO$_4$ 0.1 g, Tris 3 g adjusted to pH 7.4 with HCl, dextrose 1 g, penicillin 10^5 units, streptomycin 50 mg). Of each pool, 0.2 ml, or an equal volume of Tris-saline, was incubated for 2 hours at 38° with 0.2 ml of antibody diluted in medium 199-2-1 to give approximately 99% neutralization in the subsequent neutralization test. A parallel incubation was carried out with 0.2 ml of Tris-saline plus 0.2 ml of 199-2-1. After overnight storage at 4°, the mixture was centrifuged in a Spinco-40 rotor for 30 min at 40,000 rpm and 10°. This centrifugation did not appear to be necessary because it did not significantly affect the results of the neutralization test. The supernatant was tested for neutralizing antibody by incubating 0.1 ml with 0.1 ml of virus diluted in 199-2-1 to approximately 3 × 10⁵ focus-forming units per milliliter. After 30 min incubation, 0.1 ml of the mixture was diluted into 10 ml of cold 199-2-1. One-tenth milliliter of the dilution was then assayed for surviving virus.

Virus purification followed published procedures (Duesberg *et al.*, 1968).

Radioactive virus was prepared by addition of 5–20 μc ¹⁴C-sugars or 50–100 μc ³H-sugars to 10 ml medium of a virus-producing culture in a 10-cm plastic petri dish. Labeling was usually for 16–20 hours. The following sugars were used: D-glucosamine-¹⁴C, specific activity 52 c/mmole (New England Nuclear), D-glucosamine-³H, specific activity 1.5 c/mmole (New England Nuclear) or L-fucose-¹⁴C, specific activity 48 c/mmole (CalBiochem), D-galactose-¹⁴C, specific activity 48 c/mmole (New England Nuclear), and D-galactose-³H, specific activity 5.8 c/mmole (New England Nuclear).

Labeling of the virus with amino acids has been described (Duesberg *et al.*, 1968).

Isolation of the virus-associated glycoprotein and protein for chemical and physical analysis. Purified virus was disrupted by incubation in 0.01 M Tris HCl, pH 8.1, 2 mM EDTA, 5 mM dithiothreitol, and 1% sodium dodecyl sulfate (SDS) for 30 min at 37°. Macromolecular components of the virus were then recovered after the addition of 5% (v/v) 2 M NH₄ acetate by precipitation with 5 volumes of ethanol. After disruption of very small amounts of virus (<0.2 A₂₆₀), precipitation was facilitated by the addition of carrier protein [tobacco mosaic virus (TMV) protein or bovine serum albumin (BSA)] Carbohydrate-labeled macromolecules were pelleted by centrifugation for 10 min at 30,000 g and redissolved in 0.01 M Tris, pH 8.1, 2 mM EDTA, 5 mM dithiothreitol, 0.05 M mercaptoethanol, 10% glycerol, and 1% SDS, or in 8 M urea containing 0.01 M acetic acid and 0.05 M mercaptoethanol, depending on the purpose of the experiment.

Standard buffer consists of 0.1 M NaCl, 0.01 M Tris, pH 7.4, and 1 mM EDTA.

RESULTS

Incorporation of Radioactive Sugars in RNA Tumor Viruses

If the B-RSV(RAV-1) or SR-RSV-A was grown in chick embryo fibroblasts in the presence of uridine-³H and glucosamine-¹⁴C radioactivity of both uridine and glucosamine was found associated with purified virus. The distribution of radioactivity, optical absorbancy, and infectivity of purified SR-RSV-A in a sucrose density gradient is shown in Fig. 1. It can be seen that the

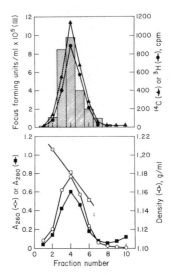

Fig. 1. Equilibrium sucrose density gradient distribution of uridine-³H and glucosamine-¹⁴C-labeled SR-RSV-A. Virus was labeled by adding to each 10-cm culture dish 10 ml of medium (Materials and Methods) containing 10 μc glucosamine-¹⁴C and 50 μc of uridine 5′ ³H (20 Ci/mmole). After incubation for about 20 hours virus was concentrated from 80 ml medium (Duesberg *et al.*, 1968) and redissolved in 0.4 ml of standard buffer (Materials and Methods). After layering over a 4.5 ml 15–55% (w/v) sucrose gradient in standard buffer, the virus solution was centrifuged for 2 hours at 50,000 rpm and 5° in Spinco SW-50 rotor and fractionated. SR-RSV-A infectivity (shaded area), trichloroacetic acid (TCA)-precipitable radioactivity, absorbance at 260 nm and 280 nm and solution density were determined on appropriate aliquots of each fraction.

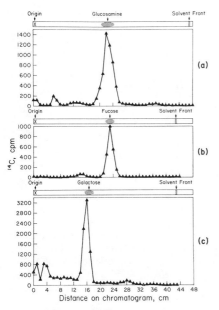

FIG. 2. Chromatography of the monosaccharide-derived radioactivity of glucosamine-¹⁴C-, fucose-¹⁴C-, or galactose-¹⁴C-labeled RSV.

(a) Glucosamine-¹⁴C-labeled SR-RSV-A virus was disrupted with sodium dodecyl sulfate (SDS), and the ethanol-precipitable material was recovered by centrifugation as described in Materials and Methods. The pellet was sealed with 300 μl of 6 N HCl and 20 μg of glucosamine HCl under N₂ in a glass vial and hydrolyzed in boiling H₂O for 6 hours. The hydrolyzate was lyophilized, redissolved in about 15 μl of H₂O, and applied to a Whatman (54 SFC) paper strip (12 × 57 cm). Descending chromatography was carried out in 1-butanol–pyridine–H₂O (6:4:3) for 8 hours (Strauss et al., 1970). After drying, the sugar spots were developed by spraying first with an acetone solution of AgNO₃ (prepared by stirring 1 ml of saturated AgNO₃ in 199 ml of acetone and adding dropwise enough H₂O for complete solubilization) and then by spraying with a solution of 5.55 ml of saturated NaOH in 195.5 ml of ethanol (Dr. C. Ballou, personal communication). The chromatograph was then cut into 1-cm slices, and radioactivity was determined in a TriCarb liquid scintillation counter by placing each slice in 10 ml of toluene-based scintillation fluid.

(b) Identification of the carbohydrate of fucose-¹⁴C-labeled B-RSV(RAV-1). Ethanol-precipitable radioactivity of SDS-disrupted fucose-

glucosamine-¹⁴C label coincides with all other physical and biological viral parameters. Between 10 and 30% of the starting infectivity was recovered after purification. This apparant loss of infectivity may be due to aggregation of the virus particles. As with the B-RSV(RAV-1) (Duesberg et al., 1968), the SR-RSV-A had a decreasing specific infectivity with decreasing buoyant density.

Addition of radioactive galactose or fucose to the medium of virus-producing cultures also led to the incorporation of radioactivity in purified virus. Likewise, purified Rauscher MLV was radioactively labeled by incorporation of radioactive glucosamine, galactose, or fucose in the culture medium.

Since all three of these sugars glucosamine, galactose, and fucose, are not, or are little, metabolized in animal cells (Strauss et al., 1970; see below), it appeared likely that RNA tumor viruses contain such sugar residues as carbohydrates rather than in a metabolized form.

Chemical Form of Glucosamine, Galactose, and Fucose in RSV

In order to determine whether the radioactive glucosamine associated with purified RSV was covalently linked to viral macromolecules, the following experiments were carried out.

1. Purified virus which was labeled with radioactive glucosamine, fucose, or galactose was heated in the presence of SDS and dithiothreitol (3 min, 100° or up to 12 hours, 36° as described in Materials and Methods) to disrupt the virus. About 80–95% of the radioactivity of disrupted virus could be precipitated with 5 volumes of ethanol or by an equal volume of 10% trichloroacetic acid, indicating that the radioactivity was incorporated in viral macromolecules.

2. Fifty per cent to 60% of the radioactivity of a solution of SDS-disrupted virus could be extracted by two consecutive

¹⁴C-labeled B-RSV(RAV-1) was recovered as described for (a). Hydrolysis was for 6 hours at 100° in 1 N HCl, and chromatography was as for (a).

(c) Chromatographic identification of the carbohydrate of galactose-¹⁴C-labeled B-RSV-(RAV-1) was carried out as described for (b).

phenol extractions and recovered from the phenol by precipitation with 5 volumes of ethanol. This suggested that most of the radioactive glucosamine was linked to protein.

The chromatograms shown in Fig. 2 indicate that almost all alcohol-precipitable radioactivity of glucosamine-^{14}C- or fucose-^{14}C-labeled virus could be recovered as glucosamine-^{14}C or fucose-^{14}C, respectively, after hydrolysis with HCl (Fig. 2a, b). About 70% of the alcohol-precipitable radioactivity of galactose-^{14}C-labeled virus was converted to free galactose by HCl-hydrolysis. The more slowly chromatographing radioactivity of galactose-^{14}C-labeled virus may be due to incomplete hydrolysis or to some cellular metabolic conversion of the galactose into other material. This is direct evidence that glucosamine-^{14}C, galactose-^{14}C, and fucose-^{14}C specifically label RSV-associated carbohydrate and are not metabolized into viral protein, RNA, or lipids.

Approximately 1.5% of the glucosamine-derived viral radioactivity was released from SR-RSV-A by incubation for 1 hour at 20° with 10 units of neuraminidase (CalBiochem) per milliliter of buffer (0.1 M NaCl, 0.01 M Tris, pH 7.4, 1 mM EDTA containing about 10–15% sucrose) without detectable loss of viral infectivity. This experiment suggests that some glucosamine is present in the virus as sialic acid.

Sedimentation Analysis of the Carbohydrate-Containing Components of RSV

Sedimentation analysis of a mixture of glucosamine-^{14}C- and amino acid-^{3}H-labeled RSV in 0.1% SDS is illustrated in Fig. 3a. The glucosamine-^{14}C-labeled material formed a peak with a sedimentation coefficient of 3.5 S based on an included 4 S yeast RNA marker (Martin and Ames, 1961). A small amount of amino acid-^{3}H-labeled protein sedimented with the carbohydrate-^{14}C material. Most of the viral ^{3}H-labeled protein

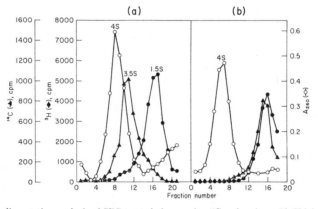

FIG. 3. Sedimentation analysis of SDS-treated glucosamine-^{14}C and amino acid-^{3}H-labeled B-RSV-(RAV-1) before (a) and after (b) digestion with pronase.

(a) A 0.15-ml aliquot of a virus solution in standard buffer containing 2 mM mercaptoethanol and 0.1% (w/v) SDS was incubated 1 hour at 37°. After the addition of 100 μg of yeast sRNA the virus was layered on a linear 10–25% (w/v) sucrose gradient in standard buffer containing 0.1% SDS. Centrifugation was for 17 hours at 20° in a Spinco SW 65 rotor at 55,000 rpm in a polyallomer tube. The gradient was then fractionated, and absorbance at 260 nm was measured after dilution of each fraction with 0.2 ml H$_2$O. Following the addition of 100 μg of yeast RNA and an equal volume of 10% TCA at 0°, TCA-precipitable radioactivity was collected and washed on Millipore filters. Dried filters were counted in toluene-based scintillation fluid in a TriCarb liquid scintillation counter.

(b) Another 0.15 ml aliquot of the virus solutions used in (a) was incubated for 10 hours at 37° with 100 μg of pronase prior to sedimentation as described for (a).

sedimented at about 1.5 S (Fig. 3a). Cosedimentation of some viral protein with the carbohydrate material is in agreement with the pherographic results shown in Figs. 5 and 11, where a minor fraction of viral protein was found to coelectrophorese with the virus-associated glucosamine-labeled material. This suggested that the glucosamine-containing material was a glycoprotein. In order to test this directly, an aliquot of the mixture of glucosamine-^{14}C- and amino acid-^{3}H-labeled RSV used in the experiment shown in Fig. 3a was incubated with pronase (Fig. 3b) and sedimented as described for Fig. 3a. The result (Fig. 3b) indicated that the sedimentation coefficient of both the glucosamine-^{14}C- and amino acid-^{3}H-labeled material was reduced to less than 1 S by incubation with pronase. It is therefore concluded that the carbohydrate-labeled material of RSV is glycoprotein It is possible,

however, that the pronase (Cal-Biochem), although it was preincubated for 2 hours at 37° without SDS, still contained substances that can degrade carbohydrate under the described conditions.

Application of milder conditions of disruption, such as by Tween 20 at pH 9.5 (Hosaka, 1968; Webster and Darlington, 1969; Tozawa et al., 1970) led to a mixture of fast sedimenting and slowly sedimenting glycoprotein material. Prior to disruption, the virus was dialyzed exhaustively against bicarbonate buffer at pH 9.5 (see Fig. 4). After addition of Tween 20 to a final concentration of 0.5 % the solution was incubated at 37° for 1 hour. Sedimentation analysis of a mixture of Tween 20-treated glucosamine-^{14}C- and amino acid-^{3}H-labeled RSV is shown in Fig. 4a. It can be seen that the glucosamine-labeled material is resolved into a fast sedimenting 8 S fraction, based on

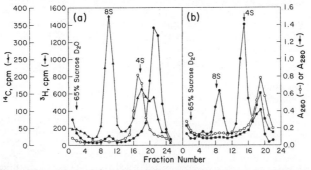

Fig. 4. Sedimentation analysis of the glycoprotein and protein released from RSV after incubation with Tween 20 at pH 9.5.

(a) A solution of glucosamine-^{14}C labeled SR-RSV-A and -amino acid-^{3}H-labeled B-RSV(RAV-1) was dialyzed at 4° against bicarbonate buffer containing 0.02 M NaHCO$_3$ adjusted to pH 9.5 with Na$_2$CO$_3$, 1 mM EDTA, and 2 mM mercaptoethanol (final volume 0.15 ml). After addition of an equal volume of a 1% (v/v) solution of Tween 20 in the same buffer, the mixture was incubated at 37° for 1 hour. The solution was then mixed with 100 μg yeast sRNA in 4 μl of H$_2$O and layered on top of a 12-ml linear (10–25%, w/v) sucrose gradient in standard buffer containing 0.1% (w/v) Tween 20. The gradient had been poured on top of a 1-ml cushion of 65% sucrose in D$_2$O containing standard buffer. Centrifugation was for 19 hours at 15° in a Spinco SW 41 rotor at 40,000 rpm. The gradient was analyzed as described for Fig. 3, but absorbance at 260 nm and at 280 nm was determined without prior dilution of each fraction.

(b) A solution containing 12 A_{260} units of purified glucosamine-^{3}H labeled SR-RSV-A containing about 120,000 cpm was dialyzed at 4° against the described bicarbonate buffer (final volume 0.9 ml). Subsequent to the addition of 1 μl of 1 M mercaptoethanol and 50 μl of 10% (v/v) Tween 20 in H$_2$O in the cold, the solution was incubated for 1 hour at 37°. After centrifugation for 5 min at 30,000 g the supernatant was collected and further centrifuged as described for (a). Radioactivity was determined from 30-μl aliquots in 5 ml of Bray's scintillation fluid.

107

an included sRNA marker, and a slowly sedimenting fraction sedimenting between 2 S and 4 S. Both the 8 S and 4-2 S glucosamine-labeled components sedimented faster than the bulk of the viral protein, but were nevertheless associated with some amino acid-^{3}H-labeled protein, suggesting that they are glycoprotein. The 8 S glycoprotein appears to be a heterologous aggregate which consists of both glycoprotein components I and II of the virus (see below) resulting from incomplete dissociation of the virus into single molecules by Tween 20 for the following reasons. Disruption of RSV by Tween 20 does not lead to complete clarification of virus solutions (see below); likewise it was previously shown that Tween 80 does not disrupt the virus at neutral pH, or does so at best poorly (Duesberg, 1970). The same virus solution, however, was completely clarified by incubation with 0.5–1 % SDS, and only slowly sedimenting 4 S to 2 S glycoproteins (as shown in Fig. 3) were obtained.

If high concentrations (about 12 A_{260}/ml) of SR-RSV-A or PR-RSV-C together with glucosamine-^{3}H-labeled SR-RSV-A or PR-RSV-C were used for disruption by Tween 20 at pH 9.5, 2–8 % of the absorbancy at 260 nm and 0.2–2 % of the radioactivity remained sedimentable by low speed centrifugation (5 min, 30,000 g), and the virus solution remained opaque. Sedimentation analysis of the supernatant is shown in Fig. 4b. It can be seen that most of the viral absorbancy had the same sedimentation coefficient as the viral protein shown in Fig. 4a of about 2 S based on an sRNA marker in a parallel gradient. The ^{3}H-glucosamine-labeled material had qualitatively the same sedimentation distribution as that shown in Fig. 4a but more of the slowly sedimenting glycoprotein was obtained. Sedimentation analysis of 12 A_{260} units of glucosamine-^{3}H-PR-RSV-C which had been disrupted by Tween 20 at pH 9.5, as described for Fig. 4b, yielded essentially the same pattern as that shown in Fig. 4b. It appeared that the ratio of the 8 S glycoprotein material to the 4-2 S material of Tween 20-disrupted virus was variable in different experiments, presumably depending on small variations of the pH (9.3–9.7), the dialysis period, and the

detergent substrate ratio of different incubation mixtures.

Polyacrylamide Gel Electrophoresis of the Glycoproteins of Different Strains of RSV and MLV

Coelectrophoresis of amino acid-^{14}C- and glucosamine-^{3}H-labeled B-RSV(RAV-1) in SDS at pH 8.1 (Fig. 5a) or amino acid-^{3}H-labeled B-RSV(RAV-1) and glucosamine-^{14}C-labeled SR-RSV-A in 8 M urea at pH 3.8 demonstrated that the glucosamine-labeled components of RSV have lower electrophoretic mobilities than the major viral proteins (RSV$_1$, RSV$_2$, and RSV$_3$). After electrophoresis in SDS at pH 8.1, the glucosamine-labeled material is resolved in a minor component I, migrating faster than BSA and a major component II with a lower electrophoretic mobility than BSA. The molecular weight of component I of the B-RSV-(RAV-1) can be estimated to be about 37,000 and the molecular weight of component II to be around 90,000 (Shapiro *et al.*, 1967) using BSA (67,000) and TMV protein (16,500) as molecular weight markers (see also Fig. 11b). It can be seen that about 10–20 % of the total radioactive viral protein coelectrophoresed with the glucosamine-labeled material in SDS at pH 8.1, as well as in 8 M urea at pH 3.8, suggesting again that the glucosamine-labeled material is glycoprotein. This was further confirmed by a complete obliteration of both the pherograms of the amino acid- and glucosamine-labeled viral components by prior incubation with pronase as described for Fig. 3b.

The pherograms of disrupted fucose-^{14}C-(Fig. 6a) or galactose-^{14}C-labeled B-RSV-(RAV-1) (Fig. 6b) were coincident regarding components I and II with those of glucosamine-^{3}H-labeled B-RSV(RAV-1). From this result it may be concluded that fucose and galactose are incorporated in the same glycoprotein species as glucosamine.

As seen in Figs. 5–11 there were small, variable amounts of carbohydrate-containing material in most virus preparations, which had lower electrophoretic mobilities than component II. The amount of this material was dependent on the radioactive precursor, i.e., there was usually more in

108

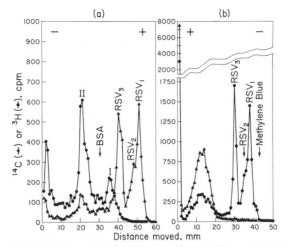

FIG. 5. Polyacrylamide gel electrophoresis of SDS-treated RSV which was labeled with radioactive glucosamine and amino acids.

(a) A mixture of glucosamine-^{3}H and amino acid-^{14}C-labeled B-RSV(RAV-1) was incubated with SDS at pH 8.1 in presence of 50 μg of bovine serum albumin (BSA) as described in Materials and Methods. The ethanol-precipitable material was redissolved by heating at 100° for 2 min in 60 μl of buffer containing 0.01 M Tris-HCl, pH 8.1, 0.05 M mercaptoethanol, 5 mM dithiothreitol, 1% (w/v) SDS, 10% (v/v) glycerol, and enough phenol red to serve as a pH indicator and tracking dye. Electrophoresis was for 4 hours at 10 V/cm in a 5% diacrylate-crosslinked polyacrylamide gel column (6 × 0.7 cm) (Duesberg et al., 1968) containing 0.1 M Tris-HCl, pH 8.1, 0.5 mM EDTA and 0.1% (w/v) SDS until the phenol red had migrated about 6 cm. Subsequent to electrophoresis, the gel was incubated for 30 min in 10% TCA until the BSA band could be located. The gel was then frozen and divided into 1-mm slices with an apparatus consisting of 1-mm spaced razor blades (Diversified Scientific Instruments, Teagarden Street, San Leandro, California) and each slice was dissolved in 150 μl of 2 M piperidine and 1 ml NCS (Nuclear Chicago) by shaking for 4–8 hours at 37°. Radioactivity was determined after the addition of 5 ml of toluene-based scintillation fluid in a TriCarb liquid scintillation counter.

(b) A mixture of glucosamine-^{14}C labeled SR-RSV-A and amino acid-^{3}H-labeled B-RSV(RAV-1) was incubated with SDS as described for (a). The ethanol-insoluble material (Materials and Methods) was redissolved in 60 μl of 10 M urea containing 0.02 M mercaptoethanol, 0.05 M mercaptoethylamine·HCl and 0.1 N acetic acid by heating at 60° for 1 min. After the addition of enough methylene blue to serve as a tracking dye, the solution was analyzed by electrophoresis in a 4% polyacrylamide gel at pH 3.8 containing 8 M urea (Duesberg et al., 1968). Subsequent to electrophoresis, the gel was fractionated for determination of radioactivity as described for (a).

galactose-labeled virus and less in glucosamine-labeled virus, and almost none of this material in fucose-labeled virus. Its presence was also dependent on the sucrose density gradient distribution of different virus preparations. If a particular virus preparation formed a sharp band at 1.16–1.18 g/ml it contained very little of the slowly migrating glycoprotein, whereas a virus preparation with more heterogeneous density distribution usually yielded more of the slowly migrating glycoprotein.

Similar pherograms were also obtained by electrophoresis of the ethanol-insoluble components of Rauscher MLV labeled with radioactive glucosamine, fucose, or galactose (Fig. 7a–c). As with the avian tumor viruses, the glycoprotein of MLV was resolved into two major components. The fast-migrating component had a relatively lower electrophoretic mobility than the minor component I associated with RSV, as seen in Fig. 7b, c, where glucosamine-^{14}C-labeled glycoprotein of PR-RSV-C was included for comparison.

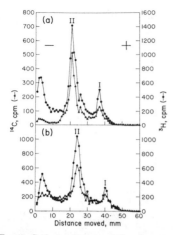

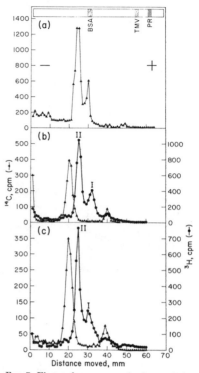

FIG. 6. Coelectrophoresis of the glycoproteins of B-RSV(RAV-1) labeled with different radioactive sugars. (a) Electropherogram of the ethanol-precipitable material of a mixture of galactose-14C-labeled and glucosamine-3H-labeled B-RSV(RAV-1) in a 5% polyacrylamide gel at pH 8.1 containing 0.1% SDS as described for Fig. 5a.

(b) Pherogram of the glycoproteins of fucose-14C-labeled and glucosamine-3H-labeled B-RSV-(RAV-1) obtained as described for (a).

It was found previously that the majority of the proteins of avian tumor viruses, belonging to different subgroups, were electrophoretically indistinguishable (Duesberg et al., 1968). These proteins were identified as components of the group-specific antigen of the avian tumor virus group. A candidate for the distinct type-specific antigens of different strains of avian tumor viruses was not detected (Duesberg et al., 1968). The search for type-specific macromolecules was now continued by comparison of the glycoproteins of different strains of avian tumor viruses by coelectrophoresis in polyacrylamide gels. If the glycoproteins of the B-RSV-(RAV-1) and SR-RSV-A, both members of the subgroup A of avian tumor viruses, were compared, a small difference between the electrophoretic mobilities of their glycoproteins was consistently detected. The major glycoprotein II of the B-RSV(RAV-1) had a little lower electrophoretic mobility than the corresponding glycoprotein of SR-RSV-A

FIG. 7. Electropherograms of the carbohydrate-containing components of Rauscher MLV compared to those of PR-RSV-C. Experimental conditions were as described for Fig. 5a.

(a) Electrophoresis of the ethanol-precipitable components of fucose-14C-labeled Rauscher MLV, which was propagated in JLS-V5 cells. The inset in (a) shows the pherographic distributions of three marker substances, phenol red (PR), tobacco mosaic virus (TMV) protein, and bovine serum albumin (BSA) in a parallel gel. BSA and TMV protein were located visually after incubation of the gel in 10% TCA for 30–60 min.

(b and c) Electrophoresis of the ethanol-precipitable components of a mixture of glucosamine-3H-labeled (b) or galactose-3H-labeled (c) Rauscher MLV, which was propagated in JLS-V9 cells, with those of glucosamine-14C-labeled PR-RSV-C.

(Fig. 8). Both viruses were grown on cells of the same embryo in the same medium, and the result was reproduced after switching the glucosamine-14C and -3H from B-RSV-(RAV-1) to SR-RSV-A, and vice versa.

110

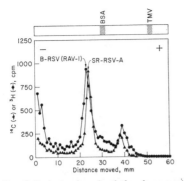

FIG. 8. Coelectrophoresis of the glycoproteins of two different strains of RSV, B-RSV(RAV-1) and SR-RSV-A, belonging to avian tumor virus subgroup A. B-RSV(RAV-1) and SR-RSV-A were propagated in different cultures of cells derived from the same embryo in the presence of glucosamine-^{14}C or -^{3}H, respectively. The ethanol-precipitable glycoproteins of an appropriate mixture of the two viruses were prepared and analyzed as described for Fig. 5a. The electrophoretic distributions of BSA and TMV protein were determined visually after precipitation with 10% TCA (cf. Figs. 5a and 7) in a parallel gel.

A more evident difference was obtained when the glycoproteins of RSV(O) and SR-RSV-A, two avian tumor viruses of different subgroups, were compared. As illustrated in Fig. 9, both glycoproteins I and II of the two viruses had different electrophoretic mobilities. In contrast to the distinct patterns of the glycoproteins of these two viruses, the majority of their structural proteins were previously shown to be indistinguishable under similar conditions of electrophoresis (Duesberg et al., 1968). Likewise the glycoprotein patterns of PR-RSV-C, a member of subgroup C of avian tumor viruses, and B-RSV(RAV-1) were found to be different (Fig. 10a). The glycoprotein peaks of PR-RSV-C, SR-RSV-A, and RSV(O) were consistently sharper than those of B-RSV(RAV-1). This may be attributed to the presence of RSV(O) (Vogt, 1967a) in the Bryan strain of RSV. The glycoprotein patterns of PR-RSV-C and RSV(O) were very similar. Only a slight displacement of the glycoprotein components could be observed (Fig. 10b), and the relative electrophoretic mobility of their major glycoprotein II was lower than that of RSV strains of subgroup A. This result is consistent with the pherograms shown in Figs. 9, 10a, and 11a where the glycoproteins of RSV(O) and PR-RSV-C were both shown to have relatively lower electrophoretic mobilities than those of B-RSV(RAV-1) and of SR-RSV-A.

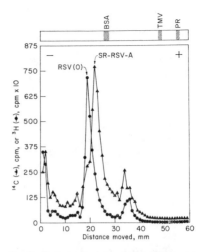

FIG. 9. Coelectrophoresis of the glycoprotein components of two strains of RSV, SR-RSV-A and RSV(O), belonging to different subgroups of the avian tumor viruses. The SR-RSV-A was propagated in C/B or C/O chicken cells in the presence of glucosamine-^{14}C. RSV(O) was grown in C/A cells in the presence of glucosamine-^{3}H. The ethanol-precipitable glycoproteins of an appropriate mixture of the two viruses were prepared and analyzed as described for Fig. 5a. The positions of the BSA and TMV protein in the pherogram were located after precipitation with 10% TCA (cf. Figs. 5a and 7) in a parallel gel. The indicated position of the phenol red (PR) marker was the same in both gels.

It follows that the glycoproteins of different types and subgroups of avian tumor viruses can have different electrophoretic behavior and possibly different molecular weights (Fig. 11b). Since the chemical structure of these glycoproteins is not known, it cannot be said whether the observed differences of their electrophoretic mobilities reflect only differences of their

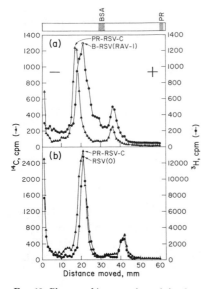

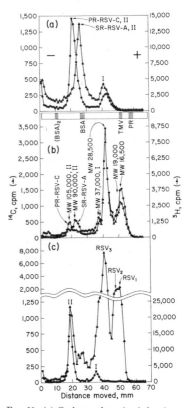

FIG. 10. Pherographic comparison of the glycoprotein components of three strains of RSV, the PR-RSV-C, the B-RSV(RAV-1) and RSV(O), belonging to different subgroups of the avian tumor virus group.

(a) Coelectrophoresis of the ethanol-precipitable material of glucosamine-³H-labeled B-RSV-(RAV-1) with that of glucosamine-¹⁴C-labeled PR-RSV-C. Electrophoresis was as described for Figs. 5a, 7, and 8.

(b) Coelectrophoresis of the glycoprotein of glucosamine-³H-labeled RSV(O) and glucosamine-¹⁴C-labeled PR-RSV-C.

FIG. 11. (a) Coelectrophoresis of the glycoproteins of glucosamine-³H-labeled PR-RSV-C and glucosamine-¹⁴C-labeled SR-RSV-A for 4 hours at 7 V/cm as described for Fig. 5a.

(b) Coelectrophoresis of the ethanol-insoluble components of amino acid-¹⁴C-labeled PR-RSV-C and amino acid-³H-labeled SR-RSV-A for 3.5 hours at 7 V/cm as described for Fig. 5a. The positions of BSA, a BSA dimer (BSA)₂, TMV protein, and phenol red (PR) were determined in a parallel gel as described for Fig. 7.

(c) Coelectrophoresis of the ethanol-insoluble material of amino acid-¹⁴C- and glucosamine-³H-labeled PR-RSV-C as described for (b).

molecular weights, as assumed for most proteins (Shapiro *et al.*, 1967).

In contrast to the obvious differences between, for example, the pherograms of the glycoproteins of PR-RSV-C and SR-RSV-A as shown in Fig. 11a, the pherograms of their major protein components RSV₁, RSV₂, and RSV₃ were indistinguishable under the same experimental conditions (Fig. 11b). This result agrees with the previous conclusion that the protein components of the group-specific antigen RSV₁, RSV₂, and RSV₃ of different avian tumor viruses are very similar or identical (Duesberg *et al.*, 1968). However, minor slowly migrating protein components (Fig. 11b) of these two

viruses were found to be different. Most of these proteins had the same electrophoretic mobilities as the glycoproteins of the corresponding viruses. This was shown directly in the case of PR-RSV-C (Fig. 11c) and B-RSV(RAV-1) (Fig. 5a), and is also indicated by a comparison of the electrophoretic distributions of the minor proteins of SR-RSV-A and PR-RSV-C in Fig. 11b with those of the corresponding viral glycoproteins in Fig. 11a. This suggests that these proteins are probably the protein part of the viral glycoproteins.

On the basis of these experiments the mass of the protein of RSV, which can be labeled with radioactive amino acids during 16–20 hours before harvesting of the virus, appears to be divided up among at least five different molecules. The proteins of the group-specific antigen, with estimated (Shapiro *et al.*, 1967) molecular weights of about 16,500 (RSV$_1$), 19,000 (RSV$_2$), and 28,500 (RSV$_3$) (Fig. 11b), comprise about 80% of the total radioactive viral protein. The glycoprotein of the virus, which includes a minor component I with an approximate molecular weight of 37,000 and a major component II with an approximate molecular weight of 90,000 in the case of SR-RSV-A and 105,000 in the

case of PR-RSV-C, comprises about 10–20% of the total radioactive protein.

Electrophoretic Analysis of the 8 S Glycoprotein Component Released from Tween 20 Treated PR-RSV-C

As demonstrated in Fig. 12, about 75% of the protein part of the 8 S glycoprotein fraction of PR-RSV-C (cf. Fig. 4) coelectrophoreses with the carbohydrate moiety, and the remaining 25% has the same electrophoretic distribution as the group-specific antigen (see Fig. 11; see also Duesberg *et al.*, 1968). [The slight displacement of the amino acid and glucosamine-derived radioactivity noticeable in component II is probably due to the different compositions of the media used to label the virus with the respective precursors (see Materials and Methods). This view was supported by additional experiments in which variation of the medium composition was found to have slight and variable effects (less than one fraction in the

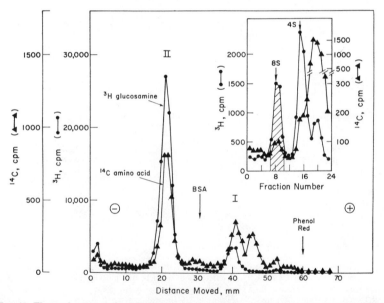

Fig. 12. Electrophoresis of the 8 S glycoprotein component of Tween 20 disrupted PR-RSV-C. A mixture of 230,000 cpm glucosamine-^{3}H and 75,000 cpm amino acid-^{14}C labeled PR-RSV-C was disrupted with Tween 20 and fractionated as described for Fig. 4. The fractions comprising the 8 S component (see inset) were pooled, and the ethanol-precipitable material was recovered in presence of TMV carrier protein (Material and Methods). Electrophoresis was as described for Fig. 5a.

gels used) on the electrophoretic mobility of the glycoproteins.] It follows from these experiments that the 8 S glycoprotein fraction of Tween 20-disrupted virus contains both viral glycoproteins I and II and some protein of the group-specific antigen. It is also possible that other viral substances, such as viral lipids, are associated with the 8 S component and that such substances might contribute to its antigenicity (see below).

Test of the Antigenicity of the Glycoproteins Associated with Avian Tumor Viruses

Two strains of RSV, SR-RSV-A and PR-RSV-C, were disrupted with Tween 20 at pH 9.5 as described for Fig. 4b and tested for type-specific antigenicity. It is already known (Tozawa et al., 1970) that a subviral type-specific antigenic component can be released from the virus under these conditions. After fractionation of 12 A_{260} units of Tween 20-disrupted SR-RSV-A by sedimentation (Fig. 4b), two glycoprotein zones were obtained. Both the fast sedimenting, (with a sedimentation coefficient of about 8 S, fractions 8 and 9, Fig. 4b), and the slowly sedimenting (with a sedimentation coefficient of 4–3 S, fractions 14, 15, and 16, Fig. 4b), glycoprotein fractions were found after dialysis against Tris-saline for 2 days to inhibit virus neutralization by chicken antibody against SR-RSV-A (Table 1), although the inhibition produced by the 4–3 S fraction was always less than that produced by the 8 S fraction. (In order to make a

TABLE 1

Inhibition of Neutralizing Antibody by Materials Released by Disrupted Virus[a]

Fraction tested[b]	Additions to virus			
	None	Antibody	Antibody preincubated with fractions from SR-RSV-A	Antibody preincubated with fractions from PR-RSV-C
Experiment 1	136, 159	1, 1		
8 S fraction			76, 82	
4–2 S fraction			26, 22	
1.5 S fraction			0, 0	
Experiment 2 (cf., Fig. 4b)	150, 173	0, 0		
10–11 S fraction (4, 5)			70, 66	
8 S fraction (8, 9)			165, 185	1, 0
6 S fraction (11, 12)			41, 58	
4 S fraction (14, 15, 16)			50, 60	5, 1
1.5 S fraction (19, 20)			0, 0	
Experiment 3[c]	162, 194	0, 0		
10–11 S fraction			3, 1	
8 S fraction			123, 114	1, 0
6 S fraction			3, 3	
4 S fraction			5, 3	1, 0
1.5 S fraction			0, 0	

[a] Data represent focus-forming units of surviving SR-RSV-A per dish; see Materials and Methods.

[b] Fractions of Experiment 1 refer to a gradient analysis of 10 A_{260} units of Tween 20-disrupted SR-RSV-A, similar to that described for Fig. 4b. Fractions of Experiment 2, containing material of 12 A_{260} units of Tween 20-disrupted SR-RSV-A, are the same as those shown in Fig. 4b, and fractions containing material derived from 12 A_{260} units of Tween 20-disrupted PR-RSV-C were obtained in a parallel experiment described in the text. Numbers in parentheses refer to fraction numbers in Fig. 4b. Fractions of Experiment 3 are the same as those of Experiment 2.

[c] Twice as much antibody was used in Experiment 3 as was used in Experiments 1 and 2.

quantitative comparison of the antigenicity of these fractions it will be necessary to determine the relationship between the amount of surviving virus and the amounts of antigen, antibody, and virus used.) Other gradient fractions, which contained some glucosamine-derived radioactivity, were also effective in inhibiting virus neutralizing antibody (Table 1). The gradient fractions (19, 20, Fig. 4b) which contained most of the viral protein, presumably the group-specific antigen, did not inhibit virus neutralization by antibody (Table 1).

The corresponding glycoprotein fractions of 12 A_{260} units of Tween 20-disrupted PR-RSV-C, however, which were prepared in the same way, did not inhibit neutralization of SR-RSV-A by anti-SR-RSV-A antibody (Table 1). This indicates that the inhibition is type-or subgroup-specific.

Since the virus neutralizing activity of chicken antibody depends on reaction with the viral surface antigen (Vogt, 1967b) and since most chicken sera fail to react with the avian tumor virus group-specific antigen (Vogt, 1967b; Armstrong, 1969), it may be concluded that the viral type- or subgroup-specific antigens sediment with the virus-associated glycoproteins.

DISCUSSION

Glycoproteins containing glucosamine, galactose, or fucose were found associated with different strains of purified RSV, as well as with Rauscher MLV. The glycoproteins of RSV consist of one major component, with an approximate molecular weight between 90,000 and 105,000 depending on the strain of RSV, and a minor, 37,000 molecular weight component. Both glycoprotein components have higher molecular weights than the components of the group-specific antigen (Figs. 5 and 11b), but appear to comprise only about 10–20% of the total radioactivity of the structural proteins of amino acid-labeled virus. The remaining 80% of the radioactivity of amino acid-labeled RSV is distributed among the coments of the group-specific antigen of avian tumor viruses. The two glycoprotein components are released in an 8 S form from Tween 20-treated virus. The 8 S form was found to be a multimeric aggregate of the two glycoprotein molecules, which was as-sociated or contaminated with a minor fraction of presumably group-specific antigen. The relative stability and biological activity (Table 1) of the 8 S glycoprotein component suggest that it may reflect the original arrangement of the glycoprotein molecules in the virus particle.

The occurrence of glycoproteins in several strains of RSV propagated on C/B, C/O, and C/A chicken cells and in MLV propagated in JLS-V5 and JLS-V9 mouse cells, indicates that the glycoproteins are specific components of the virus. The finding that glycoproteins of avian tumor viruses sediment with the type- or subgroup-specific antigens of Tween 20-disrupted virus suggests that they are associated with the outer envelope of the virus and comprise at least part of these antigens. This view is supported by the observation that the glycoproteins of serologically distinct strains of avian tumor viruses, which were grown on the same type of cells (except for RSV(O)), have different electrophoretic properties, whereas the group-specific protein components of these viruses could not be distiguished by these methods (Duesberg et al., 1968). Since the type-specific antigen is sensitive to proteolytic enzymes (Tozawa et al., 1970) and since the only protein contaminant detectable in the 8 S fraction appears to be a component of the group-specific antigen (Figs. 11 and 12), it seems unlikely that the antigenicity of these fractions is due to the presence of a minor contaminant. Further fractionation of the virus-associated glycoproteins will be needed to decide whether one or both of them are identical with the type-specific antigen.

The Friend-Moloney-Rauscher (FMR) antigen detected by a cytotoxicity assay on the surface of leukemic mouse cells has recently been isolated in a soluble form (Lilly and Nathenson, 1969). This antigen has been obtained from cells and sera and also from disrupted virus particles (Lilly, personal communication). It appears to exist in two forms, one which is larger than 7 S and the other which is smaller. This situation may be analogous to the distribution of Tween 20-released type- or subgroup-specific antigens of RSV (Fig. 4, Table 1). Since the FMR antigen is also subgroup-specific (Old and Boyse, 1965), its structure may be simi-

115

lar to the avian type- or subgroup-specific antigens and it may contain the above-described MLV-glycoproteins.

It is not yet possible to say whether the carbohydrate and protein components of the glycoproteins are specified by the viral genome, the host cell, or a combination of the two. The finding that only two of the viral proteins, probably both components of the type- or subgroup-specific antigen, contain glucosamine, galactose, or fucose, while the proteins of the group-specific antigen do not, is evidence for a specifically controlled addition of these sugars. The viral genome is probably large enough (Duesberg, 1970) to code for both the protein portion and the transferase enzymes required to add monosaccharides to it. However, a role for the host cell in carbohydrate addition is suggested by analogy with other RNA-containing animal viruses, such as Sindbis, influenza, and vesicular stomatitis viruses. These viruses, like the RNA tumor viruses, mature by budding through the cellular membranes (Fenner, 1968) which contain most of the glycoproteins of the cell (Bosmann et al., 1969). These three viruses all contain envelope glycoproteins (Strauss et al., 1970; Laver and Webster, 1966; Burge and Huang, personal communication). In the case of both Sindbis and influenza virus, it has been shown that the composition of the carbohydrate of the virus varies according to the cells on which the virus is grown (Strauss et al., 1970; Laver and Webster, 1966). The carbohydrate composition of influenza virus is very similar to that of the uninfected chick embryo allantoic membrane (Frommhagen et al., 1959). It is also possible that the viral genome could specify transferases which would synthesize the carbohydrate component in conjunction with cellular enzymes. A model for this idea is provided by the ε phages of *Salmonella*, which specify enzymes that modify the cell wall lipopolysaccharide (O-antigen) (Bray and Robbins, 1967; Losick and Robbins, 1967).

ACKNOWLEDGMENTS

The authors would like to thank Dr. H. Rubin for numerous discussions and support and Dr. W. M. Stanley for encouragement. Advice for the chemical analysis of carbohydrates by Dr. C. Ballou, Berkeley, and the gift of preprints by Drs. Strauss, Burge, Darnell, and Tozawa, Bauer, Graf, and Gelderblom, are gratefully acknowledged. We also thank Zmira Timor and Mildred Hughes for excellent technical assistance.

REFERENCES

Armstrong, D. (1969). Multiple group-specific antigen components of avian tumor viruses detected with chicken and hamster sera. *J. Virol.* **3**, 133–139.

Baluda, M. A., and Nayak, D. P. (1969). Incorporation of precursors into ribonucleic acid, protein, glycoprotein, and lipoprotein of avian myeloblastosis virions. *J. Virol.* **4**, 554–566.

Bonar, R. A., and Beard, J. W. (1959). Virus of avian myeloblastosis. XII. Chemical constitution. *J. Nat. Cancer Inst.* **23**, 183–197.

Bosmann, H. B., Hagopian, A., and Eylar, E. H. (1969). Cellular membranes: the biosynthesis of glycoprotein and glycolipid in HeLa cell membranes. *Arch. Biochem. Biophys.* **130**, 573–583.

Bray, D., and Robbins, P. W. (1967). Mechanism of ε¹⁵ conversion studied with bacteriophage mutants. *J. Mol. Biol.* **30**, 457–475.

Burge, B. W., and Strauss, J. H. (1970). Glycopeptides of the membrane glycoprotein of Sindbis virus. *J. Mol. Biol.* **47**, 449–466.

Duesberg, P. H. (1970). On the structure of RNA tumor viruses. *Curr. Top. Microbiol. Immunol.* **51**, 79–104.

Duesberg, P. H., and Robinson, W. S. (1966). Nucleic acid and proteins isolated from the Rauscher mouse leukemia virus (MLV). *Proc. Nat. Acad. Sci. U.S.* **55**, 219–227.

Duesberg, P. H., Robinson, H. L., Robinson, W. S., Huebner, R. J., and Turner, H. C. (1968). Proteins of Rous sarcoma virus. *Virology* **36**, 73–86.

Duff, R. G., and Vogt, P. K. (1969). Characteristics of two new avian tumor virus subgroups. *Virology* **39**, 18–30.

Fenner, F. (1968). The replication of riboviruses. *In* "The Biology of Animal Viruses" Vol. 1, pp. 231–277. Academic Press, New York.

Frommhagen, L. H., Knight, C. A., and Freeman, N. K. (1959). The ribonucleic acid, lipid, and polysaccharide constituents of influenza virus preparations. *Virology* **8**, 176–197.

Hosaka, Y. (1968). Isolation and structure of the nucleocapsid of HVJ. *Virology* **35**, 445–457.

Ishizaki, R., and Vogt, P. K. (1966). Immunological relationships among envelope antigens of avian tumor viruses. *Virology* **30**, 375–387.

Laver, W. G., and Webster, R. G. (1966). The structure of influenza viruses. IV. Chemical studies of the host antigen. *Virology* **30**, 104–115.

LILLY, F., and NATHENSON, S. G. (1969). Studies on the FMR antigen. *Transplant. Proc.* **1**, 85–89.

LOSICK, R., and ROBBINS, P. W. (1967). Mechanism of ε¹⁵ conversion studied with a bacterial mutant. *J. Mol. Biol.* **30**, 445–455.

MARTIN, R. G., and AMES, B. N. (1961). A method for determining the sedimentation behavior of enzymes: Application to protein mixtures. *J. Biol. Chem.* **236**, 1372–1379.

OLD, L. J., and BOYSE, E. A. (1965). Antigens of tumors and leukemias induced by viruses. *Fed. Proc.* **24**, 1009–1017.

PURCELL, R. H., BONAR, R. A., BEARD, D., and BEARD, J. W. (1962). Virus of avian myeloblastosis. XX. Amino acid composition. *J. Nat. Cancer Inst.* **28**, 1003–1011.

RUBIN, H. (1960). A virus in chick embryos which induces resistance *in vitro* to infection with Rous sarcoma virus. *Proc. Nat. Acad. Sci. U.S.* **46**, 1105–1119.

SHAPIRO, A. L., VIÑUELA, E., and MAIZEL, J. V. (1967). Molecular weight estimation of polypeptide chains by electrophoresis in SDS-polyacrylamide gels. *Biochem. Biophys. Res. Commun.* **28**, 815–820.

STRAUSS, J. H., BURGE, B. W., and DARNELL, J. E. (1970). Carbohydrate content of the membrane protein of Sindbis virus. *J. Mol, Biol.* **47**, 437–448.

TOYOSHIMA, K., and VOGT, P. K. (1969). Enhancement and inhibition of avian sarcoma viruses by polycations and polyanions. *Virology* **38**, 414–426.

TOZAWA, H., BAUER, H., GRAF, T., and GELDERBLOM, H. (1970). Strain-specific antigen of the avian leukosis sarcoma virus group. I. Isolation and immunological characterization. *Virology* **40**, 530–539.

VOGT, P. K. (1967a). A virus released by "nonproducing" Rous sarcoma cells. *Proc. Nat. Acad. Sci. U.S.* **58**, 801–808.

VOGT, P. K. (1967b). Virus-directed host responses in the avian leukosis and sarcoma complex. *In* "Perspectives in Virology" (Morris Pollard, ed.), Vol. 5, pp. 199–224. Academic Press, New York.

VOGT, P. K. (1970). Envelope classification of avian RNA tumor viruses. "The IV International Symposium on Comparative Leukemia Research" (Cherry Hill, New Jersey, September 1969). Bibliotheca Haematologica, Karger, Basel, Switzerland, in press.

VOGT, P. K., and ISHIZAKI, R. (1965). Reciprocal patterns of genetic resistance to avian tumor viruses in two lines of chickens. *Virology* **26**, 664–672.

WEBSTER, R. G., and DARLINGTON, R. W. (1969). Disruption of myxoviruses with Tween 20 and isolation of biologically active hemagglutinin and neuraminidase subunits. *J. Virol.* **4**, 182–187.

Isolation and Characterization of Proteins from Rous Sarcoma Virus[1]

PAUL P. HUNG, HARRIET L. ROBINSON, AND WILLIAM S. ROBINSON

INTRODUCTION

Ultrastructural and chemical studies indicate that the avian tumor viruses have a complex structure. An outer membrane or envelope, an intermediate membrane and an electron dense "nucleoid" have been described in electron micrographs of negatively stained virions (Bonar et al., 1963; Eckert et al., 1963). Chemical analysis has shown that protein makes up most of the dry weight of avian myeloblastosis virus (AMV), lipid 30-35% and RNA 1-2% (Bonar and Beard, 1959). Purified avian myeloblastosis virus has also been shown to

[1] This investigation was supported by U.S. Public Health Service research grant CA 10467.

contain a small amount of carbohydrate with about 1.9 moles of glucosamine per 100 moles amino acid (Bonar and Beard, 1959; Purcell et al., 1962). The detailed structure and function of the carbohydrate are unknown.

Analysis of the protein components after dissociation of viruses with sodium dodecyl sulfate (SDS) has revealed five components from AMV in Tiselius electrophoresis (Bauer and Schäfer, 1965) and three major radioactive components in the Bryan high titer strain of Rous sarcoma virus (RSV(RAV-1)) and RSV(0) labeled with radioactive amino acids separated by electrophoresis in polyacrylamide gels (Duesberg et al., 1968). Six to eight components were detected by staining polyacrylamide gels after electrophoresis

118

of AMV dissociated with Tween 80 and ether (Allen, 1967) and RSV(RAV-1) and AMV dissociated with SDS (Duesberg et al., 1968). Thus there is little agreement on the number of protein components in these viruses and little is known about the detailed structure of the proteins or their arrangement and functional role in virions.

Two antigens have been described in avian tumor viruses. The group-specific antigen which appears to be a common internal component of all avian tumor viruses reacts with serum from hamsters bearing Schmidt-Ruppin RSV induced tumors (Huebner et al., 1964). Two or more components in SDS dissociated viruses, have been shown to react with group-specific antiserum from hamsters in complement fixation (Duesberg et al., 1968) and by immunodiffusion and immunoelectrophoresis (Roth and Dougherty, 1969). A single component in AMV dissociated with SDS (Bauer and Schäfer, 1965) or with Tween 80 and ether (Allen, 1967) was found to react with a group-specific antiserum prepared by immunizing rabbits with components of dissociated virus. Further chemical characterization of the latter protein has been reported (Allen, 1968, 1969).

A second antigen in these viruses, a type-specific antigen, is thought to be on the virion surface because it reacts with virus neutralizing antiserum (Hanafusa et al., 1964). Little is known about the chemical nature of the type specific antigen although a recent report describes a component in Tween 20 disrupted avian tumor viruses which appeared to react with antibody to type specific antigens and was inactivated by proteolytic enzymes (Tozawa et al., 1970).

The present study was done to more carefully determine the number and structure of protein components in RSV(RAV-1) using methods which permitted recovery of 100% of the viral protein. When isoelectric focusing in urea as well as electrophoresis in polyacrylamide gels containing SDS were used to separate the virion components, eight proteins were identified. Only two of these were found to react in high titer by complement fixation and by immunodiffusion with hamster antiserum to gs antigen.

The three largest virion proteins were found to be glycoproteins. When virus was dissociated with a neutral detergent the glycoproteins were released from the virus in the form of a complex which was dissociated to smaller units by SDS. A separate report will give evidence that the glycoprotein components react with antiserum to the type specific virion antigen.

MATERIALS AND METHODS

Virus and radioactive virus. The Bryan high-titer strain of Rous sarcoma virus RSV(RAV-1) was grown in type C/B (Vogt and Ishizaki, 1965) chick embryo fibroblasts with growth medium 1 (Hobom-Schnegg et al., 1970). Virus was purified from large volumes of culture medium by an initial centrifugation at 10,000 g for 10 min at 2° to remove cell debris. The supernatant was then centrifuged at 19,000 rpm in the Spinco 19 rotor for 4 hr at 2°. The pellet which contained the virus was resuspended in 1/1000 the original volume of medium by pipetting and sonication in buffer containing 0.1 M NaCl, 0.01 M Tris·HCl, pH 7.5, and 0.001 M EDTA. After centrifugation at 10,000 g for 5 min, the supernatant which contained the virus was layered over a 15% to 60% sucrose density gradient as previously described (Robinson et al., 1965) and centrifuged in a Spinco SW 40 rotor at 40,000 rpm for 2 hr at 2°, at which time the virus band was collected. Radioactive virus was purified from small volumes of medium in discontinuous and linear sucrose density gradients as previously described (Duesberg et al., 1968). Radioactive RSV(RAV-1) wa prepared by incubating infected culture with a mixture of 15 ^{14}C-labeled amino acid (approximately 100 mCi/mmole, New Eng land Nuclear Corp.) or with glucosamine-[3]I (200 mCi/mmole, New England Nuclea Corp.) Cultures containing 1 to 2 × 10 transformed cells per 100 mm culture dish were incubated with 6 ml of medium composed of amino acid free medium 199, 72 parts; regular medium 199, 20 parts; tryptose phosphate broth solution, 1 part; dialyzed calf serum, 4 parts; dialyzed chicken serum, 1 part; and ^{14}C-labeled amino acid mixture to give 1.0–2.5 µCi/ml of medium. The medium was changed 4 times at 12-hr intervals, and the pooled medium samples were used for virus purification. RSV-(RAV-1) was labeled with glucosamine-³H by similar incubation of cultures with growth medium 1 (Hobom-Schnegg *et al.*, 1970) containing 15 μCi/ml glucosamine-³H.

Isoelectric focusing of virus. Isoelectric focusing was carried out in a 110-ml glass column (Model S100-10, LKB Instruments, Inc.) as described by Svensson (1962). In atypical experiments, radioactive RSV-(RAV-1) with several milligrams of carrier RSV(RAV-1) was mixed with the dense solution (33% sucrose) containing 1.9 ml of Ampholine Carrier Ampholytes (40%, LKB S141) in a total volume of 55 ml. The light solution (5% sucrose) containing 0.6 ml of the same Ampholine Carrier Ampholytes was also 55 ml and usually contained a marker protein (e.g., hemoglobin) or RSV-(RAV-1) labeled with a second isotope. The cathode solution (20 ml) in the bottom 'of the column was 60% sucrose containing 1.5% monoethanol amine. After a linear sucrose gradient was made from the dense and the light solutions, the anode solution (5 ml, 1% sulfuric acid) was layered on top of the gradient. A linear pH gradient of 3 to 10 was formed by applying 600 V for 36 hr to the column maintained at 4°. The marker protein migrated to its pI within 24 hr.

At the end of a run, approximately 60 fractions were collected from the bottom of the column. A 100-μl aliquot was taken from each fraction and mixed with 5 ml of Aquasol (New England Nuclear Corp.) for the measurement of radioactivity and pH and A_{280} determinations were made on appropriate fractions.

Dissociation of virus and isoelectric focusing of viral components. The purified virus in sucrose density gradient fractions (0.1 *M* NaCl, 0.01 *M* Tris pH 7.4, 0.001 *M* EDTA, and approximately 40–45% sucrose) was dissociated by addition of a neutral detergent, Brij 35 (Pierce Chemical Co., Rockford, Illinois) mercaptoethanol, and urea (ultra pure grade, Mann Research Labs.) to final concentrations 'of 0.1, 1.0, and 24%, respectively, followed by incubation at 37° for 30 min. Isoelectric focusing was carried out as described above except that sucrose

was replaced by urea in the dense (48% urea) and the light (24% urea) solutions to increase the protein solubility. A 50-μl aliquot was removed from each fraction to determine radioactivity.

Polyacrylamide gel-electrophoresis in sodium dodecyl sulfate. Radioactive virus labeled with either amino acid-¹⁴C or glucosamine-³H was dissociated with 1% SDS, 4 *m* urea and 1% 2-mercaptoethanol for 30 min at 37°. Horse heart cytochrome *c* (Calbiochem), 100 μg, was added as a marker. Electrophoresis was carried out in a 4 × 100 mm 7% cross-linked polyacrylamide gel containing 0.01 *m* sodium phosphate buffer pH 7.2 and 0.1% SDS (Shapiro *et al.*, 1967) for 3 hr at 10 volts per cm. The gel was frozen and cut into 1.5 mm slices. Radioactivity in each slice was measured by adding 10 ml of Aquasol to the slice after it had been shaken for 2 hr with 0.7 ml of water. Aliquots from fractions collected from electrofocusing columns were prepared for electrophoresis in SDS-gel columns by adjusting them to pH 7 with 1 *M* NaOH and adding SDS and 2-mercaptoethanol to final concentrations of 1% each. Molecular weights of viral proteins were estimated by comparing their mobilities with those of marker proteins (cytochrome *c*, chymotrypsinogen, ovalbumin, and ovalbumin dimer) as described by Shapiro *et al.* (1967).

Gel filtration of viral components. Bio-Gel P-60 or P-150 was equilibrated and washed with a phosphate buffer (0.1 *M*, pH 7.2; 0.1 *M* NaCl) before packing into a column (0.9 × 74 cm). One-milliliter aliquots from selected fractions from electrofocusing columns were chromatographed directly with the phosphate buffer using Blue dextran (Pharmacia) and cytochrome *c* as markers. One-milliliter fractions from the Biogel columns were analyzed for radioactivity by mixing an aliquot of the fraction with 10 ml of Aquasol for scintillation counting (Fig. 5).

Serum against the group-specific antigen of avian tumor viruses and complement fixation tests. Antiserum against the group-specific antigens from hamsters bearing Schmidt-Ruppin RSV-induced tumors was obtained from Flow Laboratories (Rockville, Maryland). Undiluted serum failed to neutralize RSV(RAV-1) or Schmidt-Ruppin RSV infectivity in a focus-forming assay in tissue culture. One milliliter from selected fractions from electrofocusing columns was desalted on Sephadex G-25 columns (0.9 × 20 cm) using the phosphate buffer (0.01 M, pH 7.2, 0.1 M NaCl) for elution. Protein concentrations of the desalted fractions were determined by spectrophotometry assuming that a 1 mg per milliliter protein solution gives an A_{280} reading of 1.0 with a 1 cm light path. The microcomplement fixation test was done by the method described by Huebner et al. (1964). For controls RSV-(RAV-1) and Sendai virus were dissociated with 1% SDS, 1% mercaptoethanol, and 4 M urea, and then desalted with Sephadex G-25 as described above.

Immunodiffusion method. Agar plates were obtained from Hyland Division, Travenol Laboratories. These plates contained 4 ml of agar of the following composition: Difco special Noble agar 2%, glycine 7.5%, sodium chloride 1%, with a pH of 7.2. In the center well of the agar plate, hamster serum (10 μl) was placed to diffuse against various fractions of purified viral proteins in the surrounding wells (10 μl each). Precipitation lines developed after incubating the plate at 37° for 24 hr. SDS-dissociated Sendai virus was used as control protein.

RESULTS

Isoelectric Focusing and pIs of RSV(RAV-1) and Viral Proteins

Uridine-^{3}H-labeled RSV(RAV-1) and amino acid-^{14}C-labeled RSV(RAV-1) were subjected to isoelectric focusing in the same column (Fig. 1) to assess the purity of the virus in preparations purified in sucrose density gradients. During isoelectric focusing, the viruses labeled with each isotope migrated in the pH gradient to form a single peak around pH 4 (Fig. 1). No difference in the distribution of ^{3}H and ^{14}C in the gradient was apparent. A small shoulder of radioactivity was regularly observed at pHs slightly higher than the main peak with both uridine-^{3}H and amino acid-^{14}C-labeled virus.

Next, virus was dissociated with Brij 35, a neutral detergent which preserves the surface charge of viral proteins, together with 1% mercaptoethanol and 4 M urea and fractionated by isoelectric focusing in a urea gradient. Seven radioactive peaks at pHs between 3.0 and 9.9 were distinguished (Fig. 2, Table 1). The proteins in these peaks were further characterized by polyacrylamide gel electrophoresis in SDS and by gel filtration with Bio-Gel P-60 and P-150.

Polyacrylamide Gel-Electrophoresis of Viral Proteins

RSV(RAV-1) labeled with a mixture of ^{14}C-labeled amino acids was dissociated with 1% SDS, 4 M urea and 1% 2-mercaptoethanol and placed directly on top of a polyacrylamide gel column for electrophoresis (Fig. 3). Under these conditions all radioactive material entered the gel. Seven peaks, some of which were only partially separated, are apparent in Fig. 3. The known protein components of the virus are numbered 1 to 8. Components 5 and 6 were not separated in this experiment although slight separation was achieved by electrophoresis in SDS-gels in other experiments (e.g., Fig. 7 and Robinson et al., 1970) and as will be shown subsequently, components 5 and 6 as well as 7 and 8 have distinct isoelectric points. The molecular weights of the protein components presented in Table 2 were estimated by comparing their mobilities to those of known proteins (i.e., ovalbumin dimer, ovalbumin, chymotrypsinogen, and cytochrome c as shown in Fig. 3) by the method of Shapiro et al. (1967).

In order to determine which of the eight SDS-gel electrophoresis components were present in the isoelectric focusing peaks I through VII (Fig. 2, Table 1), an aliquot of each of the peaks was made up to 1% with SDS and analyzed by SDS-gel electrophoresis using cytochrome c as a marker. The results are shown in Fig. 4 and tabulated in Table 1. Isoelectric focusing peak I (fraction 6, Fig. 2) contained SDS-gel electrophoresis protein 6 (Fig. 4a). Peak II (fraction 14, Fig. 2) contained almost exclusively protein 4 (Fig. 4b). Peak III (fraction 21, Fig. 2) contained mostly protein 8 and a

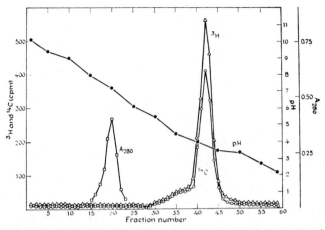

FIG. 1. Isoelectric focusing of RSV (RAV-1) labeled with ^{14}C-amino acids (O----O) and uridine-^{3}H (△——△). Approximately 30,000 cpm of ^{14}C-amino acid-labeled RSV (RAV-1) was mixed in the dense sucrose solution and 20,000 cpm uridine-^{3}H-labeled RSV (RAV-1) and hemoglobin (□——□) in the light sucrose solution, and a density gradient was formed for isoelectric focusing as described in Materials and Methods. The pH (●——●) of the fractions collected was determined after an isoelectric focusing run with 600 V at 2° for 36 hr.

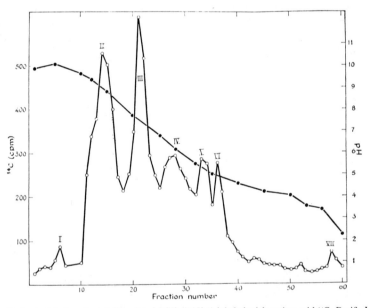

FIG. 2. Isoelectric focusing of dissociated RSV (RAV-1) labeled with amino acid-^{14}C. Purified virus (25 A_{280} units) together with 4 × 10s cpm of ^{14}C-amino acid labeled RSV (RAV-1) was dissociated with Brij 35, mercaptoethanol, and urea and isoelectric focusing was carried out as described in Materials and Methods. Two-milliliter fractions were collected and pH (●——●) and the radioactivity (O——O) in aliquots of each fraction were determined.

122

TABLE 1

RSV (RAV-1) Protein Components Separated by Isoelectric Focusing and Their Complement Fixation Reaction with Hamster Antiserum

Protein component		pI[c]	Percent of total radioactive amino acid[d]	CF-titer of a 1 mg per ml protein solution[c]
Electro-focus[a]	SDS gel electro-phoresis			
I	6	9.9	2	Negative
II	4	8.9	31	1:9300
III	8(5)	7.4	27	1:1400
IV	5, 3, 2	6.3	19	1:53
V	2(7)	5.3	9	1:39
VI	7, 1	4.9	8	1:100
VII	1, g − 4	3.5	2	Negative
Controls				
SDS-dissociated Sendai virus				Negative
SDS-dissociated RSV(RAV-1)				1:1270
Undissociated RSV (RAV-1)				Negative
Uninfected C/O chick embryo fibroblasts				1:32

[a] Peaks from isoelectric focusing column are those shown in Fig. 2.

[b] SDS gel electrophoresis components determined by the experiment shown in Fig. 4. Parentheses indicate components present in each isoelectric focusing peak in a relatively small amount and also present in much greater amounts in adjacent isoelectrofocus peaks suggesting contaminants from adjacent peak during collection.

[c, d] Data taken from Fig. 2.

[e] CF-titer were performed as described in Materials Methods.

small amount of protein 5 (Fig. 4c). The small amount of protein 5 may come from peak IV which partially overlaps peak III. Peak IV (fraction 28, Fig. 2) contained three components, proteins 2, 3, and 5, with protein 5 in the greatest amount (Fig. 4d). Comparison of the electrophoretic mobility of protein 6 (Fig. 4a) and protein 5 (Fig. 4b) with that of cytochrome c indicates that protein 5 has a slightly lower mobility than protein 6. Figure 4e shows that peak V (fraction 34, Fig. 2), contained proteins 2 and 7, protein 7 probably coming from the adjacent peak VI. Figure 4f indicates that peak VI (fraction 36, Fig. 3) contained proteins 7 and 1. Protein 7 had the same mobility as cytochrome c and was easily distinguished from protein 8 (Fig. 4c) which moved faster than cytochrome c. Peak VII

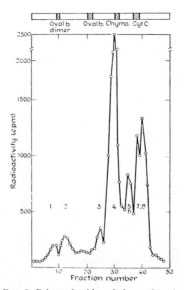

Fig. 3. Polyacrylamide gel-electrophoresis of SDS-dissociated RSV (RAV-1). Amino acid-^{14}C-labeled RSV(RAV-1) (2.8 × 10^4 cpm) was dissociated with 1% SDS, 1% mercaptoethanol, and 4 M urea at 37° for 30 min. Electrophoresis and counting of gel slices are described in Materials and Methods.

was not run because of its low radioactivity, but its characteristics will be discussed subsequently. From this experiment it is clear that the proteins of the pairs P-5 and 6 and P-7 and 8 which are not easily separated by SDS-gel electrophoresis are separate proteins with distinct isoelectric points.

Gel Filtration of Fractions from the Isoelectric Focusing Column

Gel-filtration with Bio-Gel columns provided a means for estimating the size of the amino acid-^{14}C-labeled virus components separated by isoelectric focusing after dissociation of the virus with the neutral detergent Brij 35, urea, and mercaptoethanol. Figures 5 a–f show the results of gel filtration of isoelectric focusing peaks I to VI. Bio-Gel P-60 was used for all except peaks IV and V (Figs. 5 d and e) for which Bio-Gel P-150 was used. Cytochrome c was

123

TABLE 2

RSV (RAV-1) Protein Components Separated
by SDS Polyacrylamide Gel Electrophoresis

Component, SDS gel electrophoresis[a]	pI[b]	Molecular weight, daltons[c]	Percent of total radioactive amino acid[d]	Percent of total radioactive glucosamine[e]
P1 (g1)	4.9	9.6×10^4	1.7	7
P2 (g2)	6.3, 5.3	7.5×10^4	9.5	56
P3 (g3)	6.3	3.5×10^4	6.0	15
P4	8.9	2.75×10^4	32.0	—
P5	6.3	2.1×10^4	13.4	—
P6	9.9	1.9×10^4		—
P7	4.9	1.65×10^4	26.8	—
P8	7.4	1.4×10^4		—
g4	3.5	—		6

[a] Components were determined by SDS-gel electrophoresis of amino acid-^{14}C RSV (RAV-1) as shown in Figs. 3, 4, and 7.

[b] Data taken from Fig. 2. The isoelectric points for proteins 2 and 3 are those of the complexes resulting from dissociation of virus with Brij 35, mercaptoethanol 1%, and urea 4 M.

[c] Molecular weight estimates are based on SDS-gel electrophoresis as shown in Fig. 3. It is not known how accurately the Shapiro et al. (1967) method of molecular weight determination applies to glycoproteins.

[d] Data taken from Fig. 7. The amount of radioactivity in P5 and 6 and P7 and 8 are estimated together since the proteins of these pairs overlap each other in SDS-gels electrophoresis.

[e] Data taken from Fig. 7. The relative amount of radioactive glucosamine in g4 varied from 5 to 20% in different preparations of virus. No radioactive glucosamine is present in P4, P5, P6, P7, and P8. See Figs. 7 and 9 and text.

used as a marker. Figure 5a shows that protein 6 from peak I of the isoelectric focusing column (fraction 6, Fig. 2) was very similar in size on Bio-Gel P-60 to its size after treatment with SDS (Fig. 4a). Figure 5b indicates that the protein in peak II (fraction 14, Fig. 2) was similar in size to protein 4 in SDS (Fig. 4b). Figure 5c shows that the radioactive protein in peak III (fraction 28, Fig. 2) separated into two components similar in size to SDS-gel proteins 5 and 8 (Fig. 4c). Figure 5d shows that peak IV (fraction 28, Fig. 2) contained labeled protein in a form which was excluded by Bio-

Gel P-150 (exclusion molecular weight 1.8 $\times$ 10^5) and thus was much larger in size than the protein from this peak after treatment with SDS. The excluded material was shown to be further dissociated by SDS and appeared as proteins 2 and 3 on SDS-gel electrophoresis as seen in Fig. 4d. The ^{14}C material retained by the gel in Fig. 5d corresponded in size to protein 5 as shown in Fig. 4d. Figure 5e indicates that peak V (fraction 34, Fig. 3) also contained labeled protein which was excluded by Bio-Gel P-150. This material was further dissociated by SDS and appeared as protein 2 in SDS gel electrophoresis. The ^{14}C component retained by the gel in Fig. 5e corresponded in size to protein 7. Figure 5f shows that peak VI contained a very small amount of material excluded by Bio-Gel P-60. The component retained by the gel corresponded in size to protein 7 (Fig. 4g). There was not enough radioactivity in the excluded material for further analysis. The results of these experiments indicate that SDS gel electrophoresis proteins 2 and 3 are released from virions dissociated with Brij 35, urea, and mercaptoethanol in large complex forms which are further dissociated by SDS to smaller sizes. Proteins 5–8 on the other hand are released from virions by Brij 35, urea, and mercaptoethanol in units very similar in size to those resulting from virus dissociated with SDS and mercaptoethanol.

Viral Components Containing Glucosamine

Radioactive glucosamine has been shown to be readily incorporated into avian tumor viruses in tissue culture (Baluda and Nayak, 1969; Robinson et al., 1970). Glucosamine appears to be incorporated as glucosamine into carbohydrate containing molecules in animal cells and almost none has been detected in the form of protein amino acid or in nucleic acid in the enveloped virus, Sindbis (Strauss et al., 1970). Recently we (Robinson et al., 1970) demonstrated that the radioactivity in glucosamine-^{3}H-labeled virus followed several of the protein components of RSV(0) and RAV-1 during SDS gel electrophoresis. As evidence that glucosamine-^{3}H is incorporated into RSV(RAV-1) particles, RSV(RAV-1) labeled with glu-

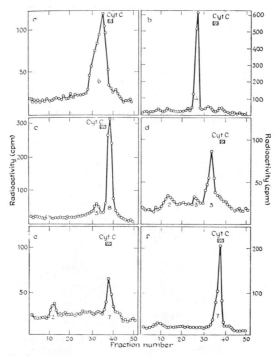

FIG. 4. Polyacrylamide gel electrophoresis of proteins in the radioactive peaks after fractionation of dissociated amino acid-^{14}C-labeled RSV (RAV-1) by isoelectric focusing. Aliquots were taken from individual fractions of the experiment shown in Fig. 2, made up to 1% with SDS and subjected to SDS gel electrophoresis as described in Materials and Methods. (a) An aliquot from fraction 6, **Fig. 2**; (b) fraction 14, Fig. 2; (c) fraction 21, Fig. 2; (d) fraction 28, Fig. 2; (e) fraction 34, Fig. 2; (f) fraction 36, Fig. 2. Cytochrome c was used as a marker for each gel electrophoresis.

cosamine-^{3}H and virus labeled with a ^{14}C amino acid mixture were purified in sucrose density gradients and then mixed and analyzed by isoelectric focusing. Figure 6 shows that the radioactivity in glucosamine-^{3}H-labeled RSV(RAV-1) coincides exactly with the radioactivity of amino acid-^{14}C-labeled RSV(RAV-1).

A mixture of glucosamine-^{3}H-labeled RSV (RAV-1) and amino acid-^{14}C-labeled RSV (RAV-1) was next dissociated with SDS, mercaptoethanol, and urea, and the components separated by SDS gel electrophoresis. Figure 7 shows the number and distribution of glucosamine-^{3}H-labeled components and their relationship to the ^{14}C-labeled viral proteins 1 to 8. Four main radioactive components designated g-1 to g-4 are shown in Fig. 7. g-1, g-2, and g-3 have the same mobilities as proteins 1, 2, and 3, respectively (Robinson et al., in press). g-4 moves with a mobility near that of cytochrome c and proteins 7 and 8. The g-4 component recovered from different virus preparations was somewhat variable in amount and in its mobility and was sometimes heterodisperse. To determine more definitely whether the glucosamine-^{3}H in components g-1, 2, 3, and 4 was associated with the protein of components P-1, 2, 3, and 7 or 8, respectively, by detergent and urea stable bonds, glucosamine-^{3}H-labeled virus was first dissociated

125

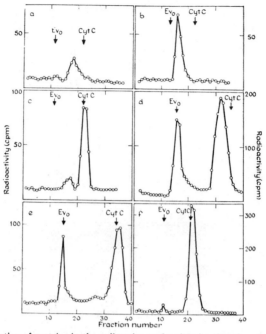

FIG. 5. Gel filtration of proteins in the radioactive peaks after fractionation of dissociated amino acid-^{14}C-labeled RSV (RAV-1) by isoelectric focusing. Aliquots were taken from individual fractions of the experiment in Fig. 2 for chromatography on Bio-Gel P-60 (a, b, c, and f) or Bio-Gel P-150 (d and e) as described in Materials and Methods. (a) An aliquot from fraction 6, Fig. 2; (b) fraction 14, Fig. 2; (c) fraction 21, Fig. 2; (d) fraction 28, Fig. 2; (e) fraction 34, Fig. 2; (f) fraction 36, Fig. 2. Cytochrome was added to each aliquot as a marker.

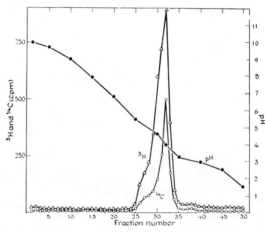

FIG. 6. Isoelectric focusing of glucosamine-^{3}H-labeled RSV (RAV-1) with amino acid-^{14}C-labeled RSV (RAV-1). Approximately 1×10^5 cpm of glucosamine-^{3}H-labeled virus was added to the dense sucrose solution and 4×10^4 cpm of amino acid-^{14}C-labeled virus and $0.4 A_{280}$ unit of carrier RSV (RAV-1) to the light sucrose solution and a density gradient was formed for isoelectric focusing as described in Materials and Methods. pH (●——●), ^{14}C (○——○), and ^{3}H (△——△) were determined on the fractions collected from the column.

126

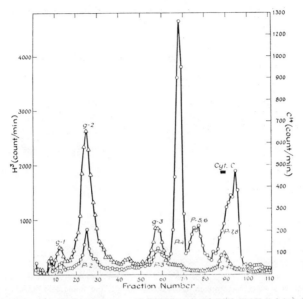

Fig. 7. Polyacrylamide gel electrophoreses of SDS-dissociated RSV (RAV-1) labeled with glucos-amine-³H and ¹⁴C-labeled amino acids. Approximately 2 × 10⁴ cpm of glucosamine-³H (△——△) labeled virus and 3 × 10⁴ cpm of amino acid-¹⁴C (O——O) labeled virus were dissociated with SDS, mercapto-ethanol, and urea and subjected to SDS-gel electrophoresis as described in Materials and Methods.

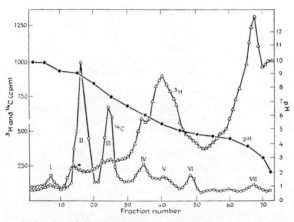

Fig. 8. Isoelectric focusing of dissociated RSV (RAV-1) labeled with glucosamine-³H and amino acid-¹⁴C. A mixture of 4.4 × 10⁵ cpm glucosamine-³H (△——△) labeled RSV (RAV-1), 2.2 × 10⁵ cpm amino acid-¹⁴C (O——O) labeled virus, 1.5 A_{280} units of carrier virus were dissociated with Brij 35 (0.1%) mercaptoethanol (1%), and urea (4 M) for 30 min at 37° and subjected to isoelectric focusing as described in Materials and Methods. Closed circles represent pH of the gradient.

127

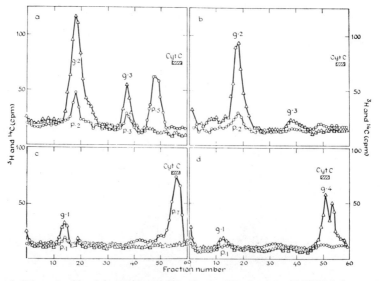

Fig. 9. Polyacrylamide gel electrophoresis of glucosamine-^{3}H and amino acid-^{14}C-labeled components from a pH gradient after fractionation of dissociated RSV (RAV-1) by isoelectric focusing. Aliquots were taken from individual fractions of the experiment shown in Fig. 8, made up to 1% with SDS and analyzed by electrophoresis in SDS containing gels as described in Materials and Methods. (a) An aliquot from fraction 34, Fig. 8; (b) fraction 39, Fig. 8; (c) fraction 48, Fig. 8; (d) fraction 66, Fig. 8. ^{14}C (O——O) and ^{3}H (△——△) were determined on the gel slices.

with Brij 35, urea, and mercaptoethanol, and the virion components were separated by isoelectric focusing and then each glucosamine-containing component was further analyzed by SDS-gel electrophoresis. Figure 8 shows the separation of components of a mixture of RSV(RAV-1) labeled with glucosamine-^{3}H and with amino acids-^{14}C. The glucosamine-^{3}H-labeled material can be seen to have a broad distribution with two major peaks at pH 5.5 and 3.5 coinciding with amino acid-labeled components V and VII, respectively, and a smaller peak at pH 6.2 corresponding to amino acid-labeled component IV. Individual fractions from the experiment in Fig. 8 were analyzed by SDS-gel electrophoresis. Figure 9a shows that the glucosamine-^{3}H-labeled material in peak IV (fraction 34, Fig. 8) separated into two components coincident with amino acid-^{14}C-labeled proteins 2 and 3. None followed ^{14}C-labeled protein 5. Figure 9b indicates

that most of the glucosamine-^{3}H-labeled material in peak V (fraction 39, Fig. 8) coincided with ^{14}C-labeled protein 2. A small amount followed protein 3. Figure 9c demonstrates that the glucosamine-^{3}H-labeled material in peak VI (fraction 48, Fig. 8) coincided with the small amount of ^{14}C-labeled protein 1 in the SDS gel. The major ^{14}C-labeled protein 7 had no associated glucosamine. The results shown in Fig. 9d indicate that most of the glucosamine-^{3}H-labeled material in peak VII (fraction 66, Fig. 8) moved with the pattern of g-4 as a heterogeneous band in the region of cytochrome c. It was not associated with either protein 7 or 8, which are found in components VI and III, respectively, after isoelectric focusing. A small amount of glucosamine-^{3}H-labeled material from VII and some amino acid-^{14}C labeled moved in the position of protein 1. When material from peaks I, II, and III (Fig. 8) were ana-

128

lyzed by SDS-gel electrophoresis, protein components 6, 4, and 8 were found to have no glucosamine-^{3}H associated with them.

These results indicate that SDS-gel protein components 1, 2, and 3 contain glucosamine and are glycoproteins. The sometimes heterodisperse glucosamine-labeled material designated g-4, although having a mobility in SDS-gel electrophoresis around that of proteins 7 and 8 is not associated with either of these protein and is thus probably protein free polysaccharide.

Reaction of RSV Proteins with Antiserum to the Group Specific Antigen

The group-specific antigenicity of individual viral components was tested by complement fixation as well as immunodiffusion using antiserum from hamsters with Schmidt-Ruppin RSV-induced tumors. Fractions from the isoelectric focusing experiment shown in Fig. 2 were passed through a Sephadex G-25 column to remove urea and Ampholyte before testing. Table 1 shows the micro complement fixation titers of each component. Peaks II and III corresponding to proteins 4 and 8 reacted strongly in the complement fixation test. Peaks IV, V, and VI had a much lower reactivity and peaks I and VII had no detectable reactivity.

Sendai virus dissociated with SDS did not react with the hamster serum. Intact RSV (RAV-1) failed to react with hamster serum unlike SDS dissociated RSV(RAV-1) which reacted at a high dilution. More than 90% of the RIF free chick embryos from Kimber Farms, Niles, California, yielded cells in tissue culture which reacted with the hamster antiserum at low titers relative to dissociated RSV(RAV-1). This low reactivity was apparently not detected in the previous study (Duesberg et al., 1968) but agrees with the findings of Dougherty and Di Stefano (1966).

To determine whether the antigens reacting with antiserum in isoelectric focusing peaks II and III were indeed different, individual viral components separated by isoelectric focusing and Bio-Gel filtration were tested against the hamster antiserum by agar gel diffusion. As shown in Fig. 10,

only protein 4 from fraction II (in well b) and protein 8 from fraction III (in well c) formed precipitation lines. Moreover, the lines crossed over completely, indicating nonidentity of the antigenic determinants of proteins 4 and 8. In agreement with the relative molecular weights of the two proteins, protein 8 diffused faster than protein 4. All the other proteins tested; i.e., proteins 5, 6, and 7, the glycoprotein aggregates from isoelectric focusing peaks V and VI which were excluded on Bio-Gel P-150 columns (Figs. 5d and 5e) as well as the dissociated Sendai virus control, did not form precipitin lines with the antiserum.

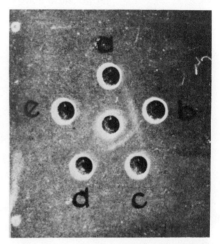

FIG. 10. Immunodiffusion of purified viral proteins against hamster serum. Viral components purified by isoelectric focusing (Fig. 2) and gel filtration (Fig. 5) were tested by immunodiffusion against the hamster serum. Serum from a hamster with a Schmidt-Ruppin RSV induced tumor was placed in the center well. Aliquots of protein from individual column fractions of the experiment shown in Fig. 5 were placed in the surrounding wells. (a) An aliquot from fraction 18 (protein 6), Fig. 5-a; (b) fraction 15 (protein 4), Fig. 5-b; (c) fraction 22 (protein 8), Fig. 5-c; (d) fraction 31 (protein 5), Fig. 5-d; (e) fraction 21 (protein 7), Fig. 5-f. No precipitin lines developed with RSV-(RAV-1) proteins 1, 2, or 3 or with dissociated Sendai virus.

129

Electrofocusing represents a method for further virus purification and assessment of virus purity after sedimentation in sucrose density gradients. Unfortunately, avian tumor viruses lose infectivity at their isoelectric point (pH 4.0) so that infectious virus cannot be recovered. Even though it is not possible to measure virus infectivity after isoelectric focusing, the fact that most of the radioactive amino acid-labeled material forms a single symmetrical peak and is indistinguishable in position from the uridine-^{3}H-labeled virus (the uridine-^{3}H was shown to be recovered in the form of viral RNA) suggests that the preparation contained little nonviral material labeled with amino acids. The isoelectric point of RSV(RAV-1) was about pH 3.9–4.0 and as shown previously avian tumor viruses with different type specific antigens are not distinguishable by isoelectric focusing (Robinson et el., 1970).

In a previous study (Duesberg et al., 1968) only three radioactive protein components were identified in RSV(RAV-1) and in other avian tumor viruses. The methods used in this study differed in several respects and permitted resolution of eight protein components. In the previous work, protein was prepared by dissociating virus with SDS, extracting the protein with phenol and precipitating it with ethanol. The precipitate was redissolved in SDS and urea for analysis. Only 60–80% of the virion protein was recovered and some was in an insoluble or aggregated form that failed to penetrate gels during electrophoresis in SDS. In this study purified virus was dissociated with SDS and urea and the whole preparation subjected to analysis by gel electrophoresis in SDS. Virus was also dissociated with the nonionic detergent Brij 35 and the components were separated by isoelectric focusing. Urea was added to the buffer system to keep the viral proteins in solution during isoelectric focusing at low ionic strength. Prepared in this way, all the radioactive viral proteins entered the gels, and 100% recoveries were made from gels and from the isoelectric focusing column. In this

study, SDS-gel electrophoresis proteins 4, 5 + 6, and 7 + 8 corresponded to components RSV-3, RSV-2, and RSV-1, respectively, in the previous study. Separating virus components by isoelectric focusing followed by SDS-gel electrophoresis which separates proteins on the basis of size or molecular weight (Shapiro et al., 1967) proved to be a powerful analytical method to separate individual viral proteins. The two methods used in sequence permitted separation of SDS-gel protein component 5 from 6 and protein 7 from 8 and these pairs were not previously separated by gel electrophoresis alone. Sequential use of isoelectric focusing followed by gel filtration which separates proteins on the basis of size permitted preparation of purified individual protein components in relatively large amounts.

Two protein components, peaks II and III in isoelectric focusing which correspond to proteins 4 and 8 in SDS gel electrophoresis, reacted in complement fixation with hamster antiserum to gs antigen. The positive reaction with these two proteins is in agreement with the previous finding (Duesberg et al., 1968) that components RSV-3 and RSV-1, prepared by preparative polyacrylamide gel electrophoresis reacted with hamster antiserum to gs antigen. However, it is now clear that one of the previously described components (RSV-1) is actually two proteins (P-7 and P-8) and only P-8 reacts in high titer in complement fixation. In addition, in this study we have shown that the other protein components in the virus react with gs antigen only at 10- to 1000-fold higher concentrations than proteins 4 and 8. These low titers of isoelectric focusing peaks IV, V, and VI may represent contamination with II and III because they trail these two during collection of the isoelectric focusing column gradient. Alternatively, the low reactivity of the protein in peaks IV, V, and VI may be specific but at a much lower titer for unknown reasons. A specific reaction with hamster serum would indicate that these antigens as well as II and III are synthesized in SR-RSV-induced tumors in hamsters.

The results of immunodiffusion with the viral components against gs antiserum indicate that II and III have distinct antigenic determinants. This is in agreement with the findings of Roth and Dougherty (1969), who showed two to four precipitin lines with SDS-dissociated viruses in immunodiffusion and immunoelectrophoresis with different hamster anti gs sera.

Components II and III are among the most basic proteins in the virion and the findings that the virus particle has a pI of 4.0 and that hamster gs antiserum fails to neutralize virus infectivity (Huebner et al., 1964) and reacts only with dissociated virus, not with intact virus (Bauer and Schäfer, 1965; Kelloff and Vogt, 1966; Payne et al., 1966; and Table 1) suggest that components II and III are not exposed at the surface of intact virions but are probably internal components. Prolonged incubation in the electrofocusing column for longer than 36 or 48 hr results in gradual breakdown of virus and the first protein components to be released were in peaks II and III (Robinson et al., 1970) suggesting that the protein components which react most strongly with hamster gs antiserum may be least tightly bound to virus particles.

The function of the gs antigen is unknown, but it is clear from this study that the highly reactive protein components 4 and 8 represent around 60 % of the radioactive protein of the virion, indicating that hamster tumors which are nonpermissive for RSV replication must synthesize at least the two proteins present in the virion in greatest amount. gs antigen is found not only in all avian tumor viruses and infected cells, but it is also commonly found in virus-free chick embryo cells (Table 1) as previously reported by Dougherty and DiStefano (1966), L. N. Payne and Chubb (1968), Weiss (1969), and Hanafusa et al. (1970). We have found relatively low titers of gs antigen in more than 90 % of the S13 line of RIF free embryos from Kimber Farms, Niles, California. Experiments are in progress to determine whether the chick embryo cell antigen is chemically identical with the virion antigen.

The glycoprotein components of RSV-(RAV-1) described here (P-1, 2, and 3) are larger than proteins P-4 to 8 after dissociation of the virus with SDS. They were recovered from virus dissociated with the neutral detergent, Brij 35, urea, and mercaptoethanol, in an even larger, complexed form which was excluded by Bio-Gel P-150 indicating a size greater than 1.8×10^5 daltons. The complex was dissociated into smaller units by SDS. This suggests that these glycoproteins may exist in the virion in such a complex. A similar complex of glycoproteins has also recently been found in RSV(RAV-1) by Duesberg et al. (1970).

The glycoproteins contain only about 5 % of the protein amino acid of the virion and their pIs are lower than the pI of most of the other virion proteins. The isoelectric point of whole virions is also lower than that of all individual protein components except for those in peak VII which contains a major portion of the glucosamine in the virus. This suggests that the glycoproteins could be surface components of the virion and account for the acidic nature of the virion surface.

RSV(RAV-1) preparations are known to consist of a mixture of Bryan high titer RSV and the leukosis virus RAV-1 (Rubin and Vogt, 1962). Focus-forming virus and leukosis or interfering virus with RAV-1 coat properties have been demonstrated in RSV(RAV-1) preparations (Rubin and Vogt, 1962; Hanafusa, 1965; Vogt, 1965). In addition RSV(RAV-1) preparations may contain particles with coat properties of RSV(0) as have been demonstrated in preparations of RSV(RAV-2) (Vogt, 1967). Previously we have shown that RAV-1 contains a relatively large amount of glycoprotein P-2 and very little or no P-1. RSVβ(0), on the other hand, was found to contain mostly P-1 and only a very small amount of P-2 (Robinson et al., 1970). This suggests that the ratio of P-1 to P-2 in the RSV(RAV-1) preparation studied here (about 1:10) may reflect the ratio of particles with RSV(0) and RAV-1 coats. Alternatively, virions containing both P-1 and P-2 in different ratios may account for the presence of both glycoproteins in RSV(RAV-1).

RSV(RAV-1) and RSV(0) differ in several properties which are thought to be determined by the virus coat. They have different host ranges, RSV(0) is not neutralized by RAV-1 neutralizing antibody and specific viral interference which is observed between antigenically similar viruses has not been demonstrated with RAV-1 and RSV(0) (Vogt, 1967; Weiss, 1967; Hanafusa and Hanafusa, 1968). RSVβ(0) also appears to infect cells with a much lower efficiency than RAV-1 and RSVα(0) has not been shown to be infectious on any cells tested (Hanafusa et al., 1970). The only known difference in coat proteins of RAV-1 and RSVβ(0) is in glycoproteins 1, 2, and 3 (Robinson et al., 1970) suggesting that these proteins may be involved in determining virus coat properties such as antigenicity, host range, interference, or infecting efficiency. Supporting this idea is our recent finding that a virion protein fraction greatly enriched in glycoproteins 1, 2, and 3 adsorbs virus neutralizing antibody and interferes with infection by viruses with homologous but not heterologous type-specific antigens. Duesberg et al. (1970) have also recently shown that a protein fraction from RSV-(RAV-1) which was greatly enriched in glycoproteins reacted with virus-neutralizing antibody.

The possible function of the other virion proteins that we have described and whether all the components are virus coded or some may be cellular proteins is not clear. Several enzymatic functions have been found to be associated with avian tumor viruses. Recently an enzyme has been described in a preparation of RSV which incorporates deoxynucleoside triphosphates into a DNA product (Temin and Mizutani, 1970), and we have subsequently confirmed the presence of the enzyme in RSV(RAV-1) preparations. In addition, RNase and ATPase activities have been found to be associated with avian tumor viruses (Mommaerts et al., 1952; Bauer and Schäfer, 1967), and these may be host cell enzymes. One or more of the proteins described here could be related to these enzymes.

ACKNOWLEDGMENTS

We are grateful to Miss Virginia Rimer and Miss Nona Stone for excellent technical assistance.

REFERENCES

ALLEN, D. W. (1967). Zone electrophoresis of the proteins of avian myeloblastosis virus. Biochim. Biophys. Acta 133, 180–183.

ALLEN, D. W. (1968). Characterization of avian leucosis group-specific antigen from avian myeloblastosis virus. Biochim. Biophys. Acta 154, 388–396.

ALLEN, D. W. (1969). The N-terminal acid of an avian leukosis group-specific antigen from avian myeloblastosis virus. Virology 38, 32–41.

BALUDA, M. A., and NAYAK, D. P. (1969). Incorporation of precursors into ribonucleic acid, protein, glycoprotein, and lipoprotein of avian myeloblastosis virions. J. Virol. 4, 554–566.

BAUER, H., and SCHÄFER, W. (1965). Isolierung eines Gruppenspezifischen Antigens aus dem Hühner-Myeloblastose-Virus (BAI-Stamm A). Z. Naturforsch. B 20, 815–817.

BAUER, H., and SCHÄFER, W. (1967). Studies on physical, chemical and antigenic properties of a chicken leukosis virus. Subviral Carcinog. Int. Symp. Viruses 1st 1966 pp. 337–352.

BONAR, R. A., and BEARD, J. W. (1959). Virus of avian myeloblastosis. XII. Chemical constitution. J. Nat. Cancer Inst. 23, 183–197.

BONAR, R. A., HEINE, U., BEARD, D., and BEARD, J. W. (1963). Virus of avian myeloblastosis (BAI strain A). XXIII. Morphology of virus and comparison with strain R (erythroblastosis). J. Nat. Cancer Inst. 30, 949–997.

DOUGHERTY, R. M., and DI STEFANO, H. S. (1966). Lack of relationship between infection with avian leukosis virus and the presence of COFAL antigen in chick embryos. Virology 29, 586–595.

DUESBERG, P. H., ROBINSON, H. L., ROBINSON, W. S., HUEBNER, R. J., and TURNER, H. C. (1968). Proteins of Rous sarcoma virus. Virology 36, 73–86.

DUESBERG, P. H., MARTIN, S., and VOGT, P. (1970). Glycoprotein components of avian and murine RNA tumor viruses. Virology 41, 631–646.

ECKERT, E. A., ROTT, R., and SCHÄFER, W. (1963). Myxovirus-like structure of avian myeloblastosis virus. Z. Naturforsch. B 18, 339–340.

HANAFUSA, H. (1965). Analysis of the defectiveness of RSV III determining influence of a new helper virus on the host range and susceptibility to interference by RSV. Virology 25, 248–255.

HANAFUSA, H., and HANAFUSA, T. (1968). Further studies on RSV production by transformed cells. Virology 34, 630–636.

HANAFUSA, H., HANAFUSA, T., and RUBIN, H. (1964). Analysis of the defectiveness of RSV. II. Specification of RSV antigenicity by helper virus. Proc. Nat. Acad. Sci. U.S. 51, 41–48.

HANAFUSA, H., MIYAMOTO, T., and HANAFUSA, T. (1970). A cell associated factor essential for formation of an infectious form of RSV. *Proc. Nat. Acad. Sci. U.S.* 66, 314–321.

HOBOM-SCHNEGG, B., ROBINSON, H. L., and ROBINSON, W. S. (1970). Replication of Rous sarcoma virus in synchronized cells. *J. Gen. Virol.* 7, 85–93.

HUEBNER, R. F., ARMSTRONG, D., OKUYAN, M., SARMA, P. S., and TURNER, H. C. (1964). Specific complement-fixing viral antigens in hamster and guinea pig tumors induced by the Schmidt-Ruppin strain of avian sarcoma. *Proc. Nat. Acad. Sci. U.S.* 51, 742–750.

KELLOFF, G., and VOGT, P. K. (1966). Localization of avian tumor virus group-specific antigen in cell and virus. *Virology* 29, 377–384.

MOMMAERTS, E. B., ECKERT, E. A., BEARD, D., SHARP, D. G., and BEARD, J. W. (1952). Dephosphorylation of ATP by concentrates of the virus of avian erythromyeloblastic leucosis. *Proc. Soc. Exp. Biol. Med.* 79, 450–455.

PAYNE, F. E., SOLOMON, J. J., and PURCHASE, H. (1966). Immunofluorescent studies of group-specific antigen of the avian sarcoma-leukosis viruses. *Proc. Nat. Acad. Sci.* 55, 341–348.

PAYNE, L. N., and CHUBB, R. C. (1968). Studies on the nature and genetic control of an antigen in normal chick embryos which reacts in the COFAL test. *J. Gen. Virol.* 3, 379–391.

PURCELL, R. H., BONAR, R. A., BEARD, D., and BEARD, J. W. (1962). Virus of avian myeloblastosis XX amino acid composition. *J. Nat. Cancer Inst.* 28, 1003–1011.

ROBINSON, W. S., PITKANEN, A., and RUBIN, H. (1965). The nucleic acid of the Bryan strain of Rous sarcoma virus: purification of the virus and isolation of the nucleic acid. *Proc. Nat. Acad. Sci. U.S.* 54, 137–144.

ROBINSON, W. S., HUNG, P., ROBINSON, H. L., and RALPH, D. (1971). The proteins of avian tumor viruses with different coat antigens. *J. Virol.*, in press.

ROTH, F. K., and DOUGHERTY, R. M. (1969). Multiple antigenic components of the group-specific antigen of the avian leukosis-sarcoma viruses. *Virology* 38, 278–284.

RUBIN, H., and VOGT, P. K. (1962). An avian leukosis virus associated with stocks of RSV. *Virology* 17, 184–194.

SHAPIRO, A. L., VIÑUELA, E., and MAIZEL, J. V. (1967). Molecular weight estimation of polypeptide chains by electrophoresis in SDS-polyacrylamide gels. *Biochem. Biophys. Res. Commun.* 28, 815–820.

STRAUSS, J. H., BURGE, B. W., and DARNELL, J. E. (1970). Carbohydrate content of the membrane protein of Sindbis virus. *J. Mol. Biol.* 47, 437–448.

SVENSSON, H. (1962). Isoelectric fractionation, analysis and characterization of ampholites in natural pH gradients. III. Description of apparatus for electrolysis in columns stabilized by density gradients and direct determination of isoelectric points. *Arch. Biochem. Biophys.*, Suppl. 1, 132–138.

TEMIN, H., and MIZUTANI, S. (1970). RNA-dependent DNA polymerase in virions of Rous sarcoma virus. *Nature (London)* 226, 1211–1213.

TOZAWA, H., BAUER, H., GRAF, T., and GELDERBLOM, H. (1970). Strain specific antigen of the avian leukosis sarcoma virus group. *Virology* 40, 530–539.

VOGT, P. K. (1965). A heterogeneity of RSV revealed by selectively resistant chick embryo cells. *Virology* 25, 237–247.

VOGT, P. K. (1967). A virus released by "nonproducing" Rous sarcoma cells. *Proc. Nat. Acad. Sci. U.S.* 58, 801–808.

VOGT, P. K., and ISHIZAKI, R. (1965). Reciprocal patterns of genetic resistance to avian tumor viruses in two lines of chickens. *Virology* 26, 664–672.

WEISS, R. A. (1967). Spontaneous virus production from "non-producing Rous sarcoma cells". *Virology* 32, 719–723.

WEISS, R. A. (1969). The host range of Bryan strain RSV synthesized in the absence of helper virus. *J. Gen. Virol.* 5, 511–528.

133

Proteins of Helper-Dependent RSV

CHRISTINA M. SCHEELE AND HIDESABURO HANAFUSA

INTRODUCTION

Recent investigations have presented a new interpretation for the mechanism of infectious virus production by the Bryan strain of Rous sarcoma virus (RSV) transformed cells which have not been exposed to avian leukosis virus (ALV) (H. Hanafusa et al., 1970; T. Hanafusa et al., 1970b). Some apparently normal chicken cells (C/O) contain a genetic element which is termed chick cell-associated helper factor (chf). Although unable to mature into a complete virus by itself, chf can complement RSV with envelope structures that chf produces in cells. Further studies have demonstrated that chf can be rescued from cells as a new ALV-type virus, RAV-60, following infection by RSV or ALV. On the other hand, chf-negative cells (C/O′) transformed by Bryan RSV produced a noninfectious form of virus called RSVβ(f−), formerly RSVβ′(O). Whether this particle was truly a helper-free Bryan RSV or produced by the assistance of another as yet unknown agent remained to be determined.

We were primarily interested in determining what differences, if any, existed in the proteins of infectious and noninfectious RSV produced in the presence and absence of chf. Moreover, earlier studies may have been complicated by the unsuspected presence of chf in C/O chicken cells. Thus we analyzed purified avian sarcoma and leukosis viruses grown in both C/O (chf+) and C/O′ (chf−) chick cells by polyacrylamide SDS-gel electrophoresis for similarities and differences in their protein patterns. We have found that the Bryan strain of RSV (B-RSV) markedly differs from the Schmidt-Ruppin strain of RSV (SR-RSV) and avian leukosis viruses in its glycoproteins.

MATERIALS AND METHODS

Cell culture and viruses. The preparation of C/O (chf+) and C/O′(chf−) tissue cultures has been described previously (Hanafusa and Hanafusa, 1968; Hanafusa, 1969). The growth and characteristics of RAV-2 and RAV-60 have also been reported (Hanafusa, 1965; T. Hanafusa et al., 1970b). In brief, cells fully susceptible to RAV-2 (subgroup B) and RAV-60 (subgroup E) were inoculated at a multiplicity of infection (m.o.i.) of 10. Infected cultures were transferred one or two times before use. SR-RSV (subgroup A) was provided by Dr. S. Kawai (Kawai and Yamamoto, 1970). The virus preparation was proved to be free of associated leukosis viruses. Transformed cells were prepared by infecting C/O′ (chf−) cultures

134

with SR-RSV at a m.o.i. of 3. The monolayers were used after one transfer.

Bryan RSVα(f+) and RSVα(f−) [formerly RSVα(O) and RSVα′(O), respectively] are noninfectious for all cell types tested thus far, even in the presence of UV-irradiated Sendai virus (UV-Sendai) (Hanafusa and Hanafusa, 1968; T. Hanafusa *et al.*, 1970a). These viruses were derived from single foci produced by infecting C/O (chf+) or C/O′ (chf−) cells with RSVα-(RAV-1). After identification of each transformed cell line as an α type based on criteria described before (Hanafusa *et al.*, 1969), the cells were grown until more than 50% of the population was transformed. Virus was then harvested every 12 hr from such cultures.

RSVβ(f−) is also noninfectious for all avian cells tested, but it can produce foci on all chick and quail cells when inoculated with UV-Sendai (T. Hanafusa *et al.*, 1970a). In this case, single foci were produced on C/O′ (chf−) cells by infection with RSVβ-(RAV-1) alone or with RSVβ(f−) plus UV-Sendai. Transformed cells derived from single foci were used in further experiments.

RSVβ(f+) [formerly RSVβ(O)] is infectious for quail and some chicken cells (Vogt, 1967; Hanafusa and Hanafusa, 1968). It is antigenically equivalent to RSVβ(RAV-60) (H. Hanafusa *et al.*, 1970). C/O (chf+) cells were infected with either RSVβ(RAV-1) alone or RSVβ(f−) plus UV-Sendai. Transformed cells derived from single foci were the source of viral preparations. Because RSVβ(f+) was grown in C/O cells resistant to RAV-60, the titer of nontransforming RAV-60 in the RSVβ(f+) preparations was always at least a 1000-fold less than that of transforming RSVβ(f+) (T. Hanafusa *et al.*, 1970a).

All of these Bryan RSVs are free from ALV, other than RAV-60 present in a small amount in RSVβ(f+) as just described above. Several preparations of each Bryan RSV type were made from single foci produced on cells of different individual embryos.

Virus purification and dissociation of viral protein. Virus for electrophoretic analysis was labeled for two successive 12-hr intervals with a L-amino acid-³H mixture (27 μCi/ml),

L-amino acid-¹⁴C mixture (2.7 μCi/ml), D-glucosamine-6-³H hydrochloride (16.6 μCi/ml; 3.6 Ci/mmole), L-fucose-³H (16.6 μCi/ml, 4.4 Ci/mmole) or D-galactose-³H (16.6 μCi/ml; 5.8 Ci/mM) (New England Nuclear, Massachusetts). Tissue culture fluids containing radioactive virus were clarified by centrifugation at 8000 g for 10 min to remove cellular debris. The supernatant fluid was applied to a discontinuous sucrose gradient consisting of 17 ml of 20% sucrose (w/w) layered over 4 ml of 60% sucrose (w/w) all in TEN buffer (0.01 M Tris, pH 7.4, 0.001 M ethylenediaminetetraacetic acid, and 0.1 M NaCl). Following centrifugation for 1.5 hr at 4° in a Spinco SW 27 rotor at 25,000 rpm, the radioactivity of the virus collected from the interface between the 20 and 60% sucrose solutions was measured. The desired fractions were pooled, diluted 2.5-fold with TEN buffer and layered over a 15–50% linear sucrose (w/w) gradient for isopycnic banding. Centrifugation was for 15 hr at 4° in a Spinco SW 27.1 rotor at 25,000 rpm. Fractions of 0.5 ml were collected, and the radioactivity of each was determined. Virus banding in the 35% sucrose region (ρ 1.16) was combined, diluted with 0.1 M sodium phosphate buffer, pH 7.2, and centrifuged for 1 hr at 4° in a Spinco Type 50 Ti rotor at 36,000 rpm. The viral pellets were dissociated in 0.1 M sodium phosphate buffer, pH 7.2, containing 1% SDS, 1% 2-mercaptoethanol and 4 M urea at 37° for 0.5 hr and then heated at 90° for 1 min. The preparations were stored at −70° for electrophoretic analysis.

Polyacrylamide SDS-gel electrophoresis. Polyacrylamide gels were prepared by the method of Summers *et al.* (1965). The gels had the following composition: 7.00% acrylamide, 0.18% N,N'-methylenebisacrylamide, 0.1% SDS, 0.5 M urea, and 0.1 M sodium phosphate buffer, pH 7.2. Polymerization was catalyzed by final concentrations of 0.05% N,N,N',N'-tetramethylethylenediamine and 0.1% ammonium persulfate. The samples containing added 10% sucrose and bromophenol blue were heated at 90° for 1 min before being applied to 11 cm gel columns in glass tubes (0.5 × 14.0 cm). The SDS-gels were preelectrophoresed at 50 V for 1 hr prior to sample application.

135

The buffer used in the electrode vessels was 0.1 M sodium phosphate, pH 7.2, containing 0.1% SDS. Since the presence of glutathione has proved to be effective in increasing the resolution of proteins (Strauss et al., 1969) 0.1 M glutathione (reduced form) was included in the electrophoresis buffer in later studies. In this respect, dithiothreitol was not as effective as 0.1 M glutathione in this study. Electrophoresis at 10 mA/gel was performed at room temperature for 5.5 hr or until the marker dye neared the end of the gel. The gels were frozen briefly before being sliced into 1 mm disks by stacked razor blades. The slices were incubated with 0.5 ml of trypsin (1 mg/ml) overnight at 37° to release the labeled proteins from the gel. Bray's (1960) scintillation solution (5.0 ml) was added, and the radioactivity of each fraction was measured. All values have been corrected for background and spillage of ^{3}H or ^{14}C.

Gel staining. Staining with amido black (0.25%) dissolved in 46% methanol containing 9% acetic acid was for 0.6 hr. Destaining was carried out in 46% methanol containing 9% acetic acid overnight.

For polysaccharide staining, the periodic acid-Schiff reaction (Zacharius and Zell, 1969) as modified by Bolognesi and Bauer (1970) was employed. The gels were fixed in 12.5% trichloroacetic acid for 0.5 hr and then placed in 3% acetic acid containing 1% periodic acid for 1 hr. The gels were washed overnight in running tap water. Basic fuchsin (0.5%) was prepared by dissolving the stain in 0.15 M HCl containing fresh 0.5% potassium metabisulfite. After stirring for 3 hr, decolorizing charcoal (1 g/100 ml) was added, and the solution was filtered. The clear faint pink stain was stored in the dark for use the next day. Staining with 0.5% basic fuchsin was for 1 hr in the dark. After three 10 min washings with fresh 0.5% potassium metabisulfite in 0.15 M HCl, the gels were rinsed with distilled water and stored in 7% acetic acid.

RESULTS

Electrophoretic Analysis of the Viral Proteins of RAV-2, RAV-60, and SR-RSV

Earlier studies on the proteins of ALVs have failed to consider the presence of chf

in C/O chick cells. Since chf can be rescued as RAV-60 by ALVs, the protein patterns formerly reported may have been distorted by this previously unidentified virus. Thus RAV-2, RAV-60, and SR-RSV grown in C/O′ (chf−) chick cells were labeled with a ^{14}C-amino acid mixture or glucosamine-^{3}H and the protein patterns compared by polyacrylamide SDS-gel electrophoresis.

As seen in Fig. 1, our findings with RAV-2 closely resemble those reported for RAV-1 (Robinson et al., 1970). The proteins are designated P1 to P8 according to Robinson et al. (1970). Peak 2 is seen only when a RSV(RAV) virus mixture is examined and thus is not present in our illustrations. The slowest migrating protein (peak 1) appears to be the major glucosamine labeled protein present. In contrast to Robinson et al. (1970), Duesberg et al. (1970), and Bolognesi and Bauer (1970), we were unable to consistently to detect a minor glycoprotein (peak 3). This suggests that peak 3 may possibly be a degradation product of peak 1 produced by the harsh dissociation procedure employing 4 M urea (Haslam et

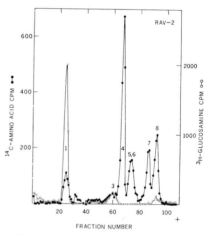

Fig. 1. Polyacrylamide SDS-gel electrophoresis of the proteins of RAV-2. Virus labeled with ^{14}C-amino acid (●—●) or glucosamine-^{3}H (○—○) was purified and dissociated as described in Materials and Methods. The viral proteins were then combined and coelectrophoresed as described in Materials and Methods. The polypeptides migrated from left to right.

al., 1970). The protein in peak 4 represents the major virus-specific protein. Although peaks 5 and 6 were not always clearly separated, the presence of 0.1 M glutathione in our system greatly increased the resolution of peaks 7 and 8. It has been previously shown that the heterodisperse glucosamine labeled material migrating from peak 7 to the anode is not specifically associated with any protein and is probably free polysaccharide (Hung *et al.*, 1971).

The proteins of RAV-60 and SR-RSV (Figs. 2 and 3) did not differ essentially from those of RAV-2. Peak 4 was again the major virus-specific protein. Polypeptides 7 and 8 were easily distinguishable, but peaks 5 and 6 remained inseparable. The low molecular weight material between peak 8 and the anode appears to be due to the included marker dye. While the minor glycoprotein (peak 3) was not distinct, the single high molecular weight glycoprotein (peak 1) was readily demonstrable. The primary difference between RAV-60, RAV-2 and SR-RSV resides in the mobility of the major glycoprotein.

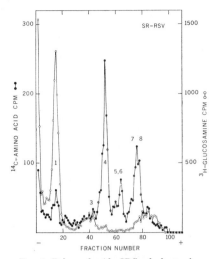

FIG. 3. Polyacrylamide SDS-gel electrophoresis of the proteins of SR-RSV. Procedure was identical to Fig. 1.

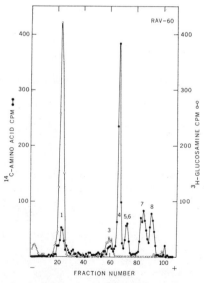

FIG. 2. Polyacrylamide SDS-gel electrophoresis of the proteins of RAV-60. Procedure was identical to Fig. 1.

RAV-2 grown in C/O (chf+) cells did not differ remarkably from RAV-2 grown in C/O′ (chf−). It was noted, however, that peak 1 was considerably broader. This could be attributed to the activation of chf to RAV-60 by RAV-2 in C/O (chf+) cells. Thus the major glycoprotein of RAV-2 grown in C/O (chf+) cells could be a mixture of peak 1 from RAV-2 and peak 1 from RAV-60. These components could appear as a single element because of their similar, but not identical, electrophoretic mobilities.

Electrophoretic Analysis of the Viral Proteins of Bryan RSV

Bryan RSV produced in the absence of ALV differed substantially from SR-RSV, RAV-60, and RAV-2. The electropherogram of RSVβ(f+) presented in Fig. 4 shows that the major change occurs in the glycoproteins. At least three distinct glucosamine labeled peaks were reproducibly demonstrated with all of several different RSVβ(f+) preparations examined. Moreover, the same pattern as that obtained with labeled glucosamine was also found when radioactive galactose or fucose were used as

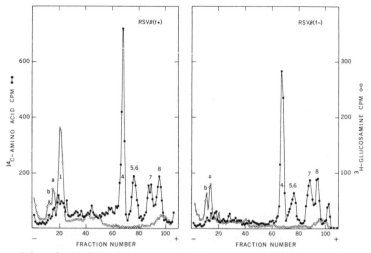

Fig. 4. Polyacrylamide SDS-gel electrophoresis of the proteins of RSVβ(f+) and RSVβ(f −) of the Bryan strain of RSV. Procedure was identical to Fig. 1.

labeling compounds. In contrast to the major glycoprotein (peak 1) of RAV and SR-RSV, the three peaks of RSVβ(f+) labeled with isotopic carbohydrates appeared poorly labeled with radioactive amino acids. However, the multiple, slowly migrating peaks disappeared when glucosamine-³H-labeled RSV was treated with pronase (200 μg/ml at 37° for 0.5 hr). This suggests that the material observed by glucosamine labeling is indeed carbohydrate-containing polypeptide even though the corresponding protein moieties are not clearly evident with amino acid labeling.

As seen in Table 1, peak 1 of RSVβ(f+) accounted for approximately 4.9% of the total radioactivity incorporated in contrast to the average 9.5% found in SR-RSV, RAV-2, and RAV-60. This apparent reduction could be attributed to the distribution of the amino acid label among several glycoproteins (peak 1, a and b) rather than a single polypeptide as seen in the other avian sarcoma and leukosis viruses. On the other hand, protein P-1 of RSVβ(f+) may be enriched in amino acids poorly represented in the reconstituted protein hydrolyzate used for labeling.

To assure that the amount of the com-

ponents present in the region of the slowly migrating glycoproteins was indeed low, a more highly labeled sample of RSVβ(f+) was analyzed. The results confirmed the previous one: Instead of a clear single protein of low electrophoretic mobility (peak 1) like that found in SR-RSV, RAV-60, or RAV-2, at least three proteins which contained smaller amounts of labeled amino acid appeared in the positions corresponding to the three glucosamine labeled peaks.

To test the possibility that Bryan RSV-infected cells contained a large pool of high molecular weight proteins which turned over very slowly, virus obtained after labeling cultures continuously for 3 days was examined by polyacrylamide SDS-gel electrophoresis. A significant increase was not demonstrated in the percentage of amino acid incorporated into the proteins of low electrophoretic mobility of RSVβ(f+) or RSVβ(f−).

The protein profile of RSVβ(f−) obtained from C/O′ (chf−) chick cells is also shown in Fig. 4. No significant differences from those previously described were found in the virus-specific polypeptides (4 to 8) having a fast electrophoretic mobility. However, the glycoproteins of RSVβ(f−) are

TABLE 1

PERCENTAGE DISTRIBUTION OF RADIOACTIVE AMINO ACID IN ALV AND RSV[a]

Protein	Viruses					
	RAV-2	RAV-60	SR-RSV	RSVβ(f+)	RSVβ(f−)	RSVα(f+)
C	—	—	—	—	—	0.8
B	—	—	—	1.3	3.9	0.8
A	—	—	—	2.4	3.6	3.3
P-1	8.7	9.8	9.6	4.9	—	2.8
P-3[b]	4.3	4.0	4.7	2.0	4.2	2.7
P-4	35.6	41.8	44.1	39.5	37.3	32.1
P-5, 6	18.8	10.2	10.7	16.9	17.2	16.7
P-7	13.5	17.9	14.2	14.4	16.2	20.8
P-8	19.2	16.0	18.2	15.3	17.0	20.0

[a] Although these values are averages of 2–5 separate determinations, except RSVα(f+), which is based on a single experiment, the percentages are only approximate due to variability in the separation of the proteins and the total amount of radioactivity analyzed.

[b] Calculated by estimating the position of peak 3 and arbitrarily totaling the counts present in the region.

reduced both in number of species and total quantity of label as compared to RSVβ(f+): The most obvious alteration is the absence of peak 1.

Figure 5 illustrates that RSVα(f+) has even more heterogeneous glycoproteins than RSVβ(f+). Otherwise, the major viral proteins are similar to SR-RSV, RAV-60, and RAV-2. Again to establish the presence or absence of a large protein, a more highly labeled preparation of RSVα(f+) was examined, and no single polypeptide of low electrophoretic mobility was demonstrable. Table 1 summarizes our findings on the percentage distribution of the viral proteins of B-RSV and ALVs.

Staining of the Proteins of RAV and RSV

The major peaks identified in the electropherograms were all also visible by staining the gels with amido black. In fact, in all samples examined more proteins were revealed by staining than by electrophoretic analysis of radioactively labeled virus. About four minor protein staining bands appeared between electrophoretic peaks 1 and 4. No clear-cut differences between RAV-2 grown in C/O versus C/O′ cells could be distinguished. However, RSVβ(f+) and RSVβ-(f−) differed from each other and from RAV-2. More bands were visible in the glycoprotein region of RSVβ(f+) and

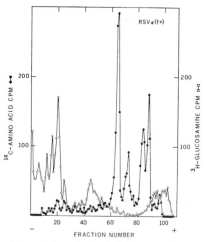

FIG. 5. Polyacrylamide SDS-gel electrophoresis of the proteins of Bryan RSVα(f+). Procedure was identical to Fig. 1.

RSVβ(f−) as compared to RAV-2. In addition, peak 4 of RSVβ(f+) and RSVβ(f−) appeared as two lightly stained bands rather than a single intense band as observed in RAV-2. Peak 3 was not evident in RAV-2, RSVβ(f+) or RSVβ(f−). RSVβ(f−) was lacking a band present in the glycoprotein region of RSVβ(f+).

To confirm the difference between B-RSV

139

and RAV in amido black staining and in incorporation of radioactive sugars, gels were stained for carbohydrate by the periodic acid-Schiff reaction. Since the glycoprotein region of RSVβ(f+) and RSVβ(f−) stained heterogeneously, we were unable to clearly distinguish any distinctive differences between these two viruses. However, RAV-2 clearly contained only one glycoprotein staining region in contrast to the multiplicity observed with Bryan RSV. No staining in the area of peak 3 was detected with any of the viruses examined.

Comparison of the Mobility of the Glycoproteins of RAV and RSV

The glycoprotein components of ALVs with different type-specific antigens have different mobilities in polyacrylamide SDS-gel electrophoresis (Duesberg et al., 1970; Robinson et al., 1970). Since SR-RSV, RAV-60, and RAV-2 all contained a single glycoprotein, the mobility of this protein was compared. Figure 6A demonstrates that, although the glycoproteins of RAV-2 and RAV-60 are closely similar, they are not identical. This was confirmed also by co-electrophoresis of glucosamine-³H-labeled RAV-2 protein with amino acid-¹⁴C-labeled RAV-60 protein. On the other hand, the

glycoprotein of SR-RSV had a mobility similar to that of RAV-60 (Fig. 6B).

We have shown that B-RSVs differ from SR-RSV, RAV-60, and RAV-2 primarily in their glycoproteins. But it is known that RSVβ(f+) and RAV-60 are closely related antigenically and perhaps have the same envelope antigen (T. Hanafusa et al., 1970b). Figure 7 demonstrates that the mobility of peak 1 of RSVβ(f+) is not precisely identical to that of the major glycoprotein of RAV-60. This indicates that antigenically similar viruses could have glycoproteins of different mobilities. It seems likely that the presence of peak 1 in RSVβ(f+) and its absence in RSVβ(f−) may account for the difference in infectivity of the two virus particles for certain cells.

RSVα(f−) is similar to RSVβ(f−) in that both are noninfectious forms of Bryan RSV. Like RSVβ(f−), peak 1 is also missing from RSVα(f−) obtained from C/O′ (chf−) chick cells (Fig. 7). This supports the idea that Bryan RSV cannot form glycoprotein P-1 without the assistance of chf or ALV. However, RSVα(f+) which possesses peak 1 is also noninfectious. But RSVα(f+) has

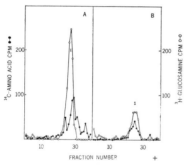

Fig. 6. Comparison of the glycoproteins of RAV-2, RAV-60, and SR-RSV. (A) Polyacrylamide SDS-gel electrophoresis of the proteins of ¹⁴C-amino acid labeled RAV-2 (●—●) and glucosamine-³H labeled RAV-60 (○—○). (B) Polyacrylamide SDS-gel electrophoresis of the proteins of ¹⁴C-amino acid labeled RAV-60 (●—●) and glucosamine-³H labeled SR-RSV (○—○). Only the cathodal end of the gels are presented.

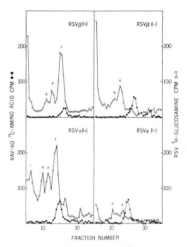

Fig. 7. Comparison of the glycoproteins of Bryan RSV and RAV-60. Glucosamine-³H-labeled B-RSV (○—○) and ¹⁴C-amino acid labeled RAV-60 (●—●) were subjected to coelectrophoresis. Only the cathodal end of the gels are presented.

been shown to lack DNA polymerase activity (Hanafusa and Hanafusa, 1971). Thus RSVα(f−) may have two virion deficiencies —one in DNA polymerase activity and the other in the absence of glycoprotein P-1.

DISCUSSION

RAV-2, RAV-60, and SR-RSV grown in C/O (chf+) and C/O′ (chf−) chicken cells all contained at least seven proteins. Six polypeptides appeared unchanged with different strains of virus in both their mobility and relative quantity. One protein of low electrophoretic mobility was identified as the major glycoprotein of the virus, and its mobility varied with the virus strain. In the present studies, the mobility of P-1 of RAV-2 (subgroup B) was greater than that of SR-RSV (subgroup A) and RAV-60 (subgroup E). The latter two P-1s both moved about the same distance. Duesberg et al. (1970) have pointed out that two subgroup A viruses, SR-RSV and RSV(RAV-1), have a small but consistent difference in the P-1 protein. We have also found that the P-1 proteins of two subgroup E viruses migrate at slightly different rates. Thus although the electrophoretic mobility of a protein may be used as a marker to distinguish two different virus strains, there appears as yet to be no definitive rule regarding subgroup classification.

The results with Bryan RSV produced from C/O and C/O′ cells without superinfecting ALV showed a significant alteration in the glycoprotein pattern. The change was characterized both by a relatively small quantity of protein demonstrable in the glycoproteins and by an appearance of multiple peaks containing the carbohydrate label. The unique pattern obtained in this study is different from that obtained with RSV(O) [equivalent to RSVβ(f+)] by Robinson et al. (1970). The reason for this discrepancy is not immediately clear. One could explain this difference by assuming that two different types of host cells were used to prepare the RSVβ(f+). We have previously described the production of RAV-60 by infecting C/O cells with RSVβ(f+) or ALV. However, the amount of RAV-60 recoverable from C/O cells, which are resistant to RSVβ(f+) or subgroup E viruses, is generally one thousandth that of the virus used for the rescue (T. Hanafusa et al. 1970). The titer of RAV-60 increases to a level comparable to that of the activating virus only when the rescue is made in C/O cells susceptible to subgroup E or when the RAV-60 recovered is passaged in cells susceptible to subgroup E. Therefore, if RSVβ-(f+) or ALV were obtained from C/O cells susceptible to subgroup E or if these viruses were passaged in cells susceptible to subgroup E, the concentration of RAV-60 in these virus preparations becomes significantly high and affects the protein profile of these viruses. Although this is one possible explanation for the observed discrepancy of RSVβ(f+) from the pattern obtained by Robinson et al. (1970), others such as mutational changes in Bryan RSV could also be invoked.

Among the avian tumor viruses examined, no difference was found in the major detectable protein components except in the glycoprotein. Duesberg et al. (1968) and Hung et al. (1971) have shown that the activity of the group-specific (gs) antigen is associated with two proteins, peak 4 and peak 8. We have found that all avian tumor viruses, including RSVα and RSVβ, contain gs-antigen regardless of the cells [C/O (chf+) or C/O′ (chf−)] in which they have been grown. We have also demonstrated that RSVα has no functionally active DNA polymerase in the particles (Hanafusa and Hanafusa, 1971). And yet no gross difference in the protein pattern between RSVα and RSVβ exists. This indicates that the enzymatic protein is either a minor viral component undetectable by the techniques employed or else present in RSVα in a form indistinguishable from the active enzyme.

The multiplicity of the carbohydrate containing peaks in Bryan RSV viruses is a subject for future work. It is conceivable, however, that this characteristic feature is a reflection of the helper-dependent nature of Bryan RSV. For example, Bryan RSV may be deficient in the formation of either a single polypeptide or the carbohydrate that is generally utilized for glycoprotein in the viral envelope. If virus were produced in the

141

absence of chf or ALV [as is $RSV\beta(f-)$ or $RSV\alpha(f-)$], a proper carbohydrate may not be available or a carbohydrate component may not be properly assembled as glycoprotein and result in the absence of a major glycoprotein in these viruses. If, however, Bryan RSV [$RSV\beta(f+)$ or $RSV\alpha(f+)$] were grown in chf positive cells, where all of the envelope components were available, then RSV would be able to form a major carbohydrate containing polypeptide. Alternatively, the defect could reside in an improper processing, such as faulty cleavage, of a correct precursor glycoprotein which may be partially represented by peaks a and b.

Although one cannot exclude that peak a or b in $RSV\beta(f-)$ functions as an envelope component in a way similar to peak 1 of other RSV or ALV, the correlation of the presence or absence of peak 1 in infectious $RSV\beta(f+)$ and noninfectious $RSV\beta(f-)$ suggests that peak 1 is a viral structural component essential for infectivity. For a long time, the failure of Bryan RSV to produce infectious progeny has been attributed to its inability to synthesize antigenic component(s) of the viral envelope (H. Hanafusa *et al.*, 1964, Hanafusa, 1965). The absence of peak 1 in the protein pattern of $RSV\beta(f-)$ could be the first physical verification of this hypothesis.

ACKNOWLEDGMENT

The authors wish to thank Susan Zanger and Lucy DiMauro for their excellent technical assistance. This work was supported by U. S. Public Health Service research grant CA-08747 from the National Cancer Institute. CMS was supported by Damon Runyon Cancer Research Fellowship DRF-575.

REFERENCES

Bolognesi, D. P., and Bauer, H. (1970). Polypeptides of avian RNA tumor viruses. I. Isolation and physical and chemical analysis. *Virology* 42, 1097–1112.

Bray, G. A. (1960). A simple efficient liquid scintillator for counting aqueous solutions in a liquid scintillation counter. *Anal. Biochem.* 1, 279–285.

Duesberg, P. H., Martin, G. S., and Vogt, P. K. (1970). Glycoprotein components of avian and murine RNA tumor viruses. *Virology* 41, 631–646.

Hanafusa, H. (1965). Analysis of the defectiveness of Rous sarcoma virus. III. Determining influence of a new helper virus on the host range and susceptibility to interference of RSV. *Virology* 25, 248–255.

Hanafusa, H. (1969). Rapid transformation of cells by Rous sarcoma virus. *Proc. Nat. Acad. Sci. U. S.* 63, 318–325.

Hanafusa, H., and Hanafusa, T. (1968). Further studies on RSV production from transformed cells. *Virology* 34, 630–636.

Hanafusa, H., and Hanafusa, T. (1971). Noninfectious RSV deficient in DNA polymerase. *Virology* 43, 313–316.

Hanafusa, H., Hanafusa, T., and Rubin, H. (1964). Analysis of the defectiveness of Rous sarcoma virus. II. Specification of RSV antigenicity by helper virus. *Proc. Nat. Acad. Sci. U. S.* 51, 41–48.

Hanafusa, H., Hanafusa, T., and Miyamoto, T. (1969). Two origins for formation of non-infectious virus from Rous sarcoma cells. *In* "Defectiveness, Rescue and Stimulation of Oncogenic Viruses" (Centre National de la Recherche Scientifique, ed.), pp. 195–199. Second International Symposium on Tumor Viruses, Royaumont.

Hanafusa, H., Miyamoto, T., and Hanafusa, T. (1970). A cell-associated factor essential for formation of an infectious form of Rous sarcoma virus. *Proc. Nat. Acad. Sci. U. S.* 66, 314–321.

Hanafusa, T., Miyamoto, T., and Hanafusa, H. (1970a). A type of chick embryo cell that fails to support formation of infectious RSV. *Virology* 40, 55–64.

Hanafusa, T., Hanafusa, H., and Miyamoto, T. (1970b). Recovery of a new virus from apparently normal chick cells by infection with avian tumor viruses. *Proc. Natl. Acad. Sci. U. S.* 67, 1797–1803.

Haslam, E. A., Hampson, A. W., Egan, J. E., and White, D. O. (1970). The polypeptides of influenza virus. II. Interpretation of polyacrylamide gel electrophoresis patterns. *Virology* 42, 555–565.

Hung, P. P., Robinson, H. L., and Robinson, W. S. (1971). Isolation and characterization of proteins from Rous sarcoma virus. *Virology* 43, 251–266.

Kawai, S., and Yamamoto, T. (1970). Isolation of different kinds of non-virus producing cells transformed by Schmidt-Ruppin strain (subgroup A) of Rous sarcoma virus. *Jap. J. Exp. Med.* 40, 243–256.

Robinson, W. S., Hung, P., Robinson, H. L., and Ralph, D. (1970). Proteins of avian tumor viruses with different coat antigens. *J. Virol.* **6**, 695–698.

STRAUSS, J. H., BURGE, B. W., and DARNELL, J. E. (1969). Sindbis virus infection of chick and hamster cells: Synthesis of virus specific proteins. *Virology* **37**, 367–376.

SUMMERS, D. F., MAIZEL, J. V., and DARNELL, J. E. (1965). Evidence for virus-specific non-capsid proteins in poliovirus-infected Hela cells. *Proc. Nat. Acad. Sci. U. S.* **54**, 505–513.

VOGT, P. K. (1967). A virus released by "non-producing" Rous sarcoma cells. *Proc. Nat. Acad. Sci. U. S.* **58**, 801–808.

ZACHARIUS, R. M., and ZELL, E. (1969). Glyco-protein staining following electrophoresis on acrylamide gels. *Anal. Biochem.* **30**, 148–152.

IMMUNOLOGICAL CORRELATES

A Cl-Fixation Method for the Measurement of Chicken Anti-Viral Antibody

R. L. Stolfi, Ruth A. Fugmann, J. J. Jensen and M. M. Sigel

INTRODUCTION

The failure of chicken antibody to activate the first component (Cl) of guinea-pig complement (Benson, Brumfield and Pomeroy, 1961; Brumfield, Benson and Pomeroy, 1961; Okazaki, Purchase, Fredrickson and Burmester, 1962; Rose and Orlans, 1962a), as well as the marked anticomplementary activity of heated chicken serum (Benson *et al.*, 1961; Brumfield *et al.*, 1961; Okazaki *et al.*, 1962; Rose and Orlans, 1962a, b; Rice, 1947; Orlans, Rose and Clapp, 1962), have hampered the development of a satisfactory complement-fixation test for the measurement of chicken antibody. For the titration of certain chicken antiviral sera, such as anti-Rous sarcoma virus, only time consuming and expensive neutralization methods are presently available.

The present communication describes the development of a sensitive method for the measurement of chicken Cl and its subsequent utilization in a Cl-fixation test for titrating antibodies in chicken sera to influenza virus and to the Bryan strain of Rous sarcoma virus.

EXPERIMENTAL METHODS

Antisera

1. *Sensitizing antibody.* Adult Kimber chickens received eight equal intravenous injections containing a total of $1 \cdot 8 \times 10^{10}$ washed sheep erythrocytes over a 3-week period of time, and were bled 2 weeks after the last injection.

2. *Antibody to PR8 virus.* 2-week-old Kimber chickens were inoculated on day 0 and on day 15 with 2 ml of A influenza virus strain PR8 (PR8 virus) which had been harvested as allantoic fluid, and adsorbed to and eluded from guinea-pig red cells. The chickens were bled at 5-day intervals beginning at day 0.

3. *Antibody to Rous sarcoma virus.* Antisera to the Bryan strain of Rous sarcoma virus (RSV–RAV 1) were obtained from Kimber chickens bearing Rous sarcomas induced by this virus.

Buffer solutions

1. GVB^{++}. Gelatin Veronal buffer with Ca^{++} and Mg^{++} consisted of isotonic Veronal buffer containing 0·1 per cent gelatin, 0·00015 M Ca^{++} and 0·0005 M Mg^{++}, pH 7·4 ($I = 0·15$).

2. $DGVB^{++}$. Dextrose gelatin Veronal buffer with Ca^{++} and Mg^{++} was prepared by mixing equal volumes of 5 per cent dextrose in water and a gelatin Veronal buffer containing twice the usual amounts of Ca^{++}, Mg^{++} and gelatin ($I = 0·075$).

3. DG^{++}. Dextrose gelatin with Ca^{++} and Mg^{++} consisted of 5 per cent dextrose in water with 0·1 per cent gelatin, 0·00015 M Ca^{++} and 0·0005 M Mg^{++}.

Sensitized sheep erythrocytes (EAb^{ch})

Washed sheep erythrocytes (1×10^9/ml) in 0·01 M isotonic sodium ethylenediamine-tetraacetate (EDTA) in gelatin Veronal buffer without Ca^{++} and Mg^{++} were sensitized with an equal volume of unheated chicken antiserum diluted 1:60 in the same buffer (10 haemagglutinating doses) at room temperature for 20 minutes. The EAb^{ch} were then washed and resuspended to 1×10^8/ml in $DGVB^{++}$ for use, unless otherwise noted. One haemagglutinating dose is defined as the concentration of antibody which produces partial (2^+) agglutination of the concentration of sheep cells used for sensitization.

Guinea-pig supernatant I (Sup. I)

A reagent containing eight components of guinea-pig complement was prepared by precipitation and removal of C1 from guinea-pig serum by lowering the ionic strength to $I = 0·04$ with water at pH 7·5 (Nelson, 1961; Nelson, Jensen, Gigli, and Tamura 1966). The resultant supernatant fluid (Sup. I) contained less than 1 per cent of the C1 activity of whole serum, but retained greater than 99 per cent of the activity of each of the remaining eight components of guinea-pig complement.

Sucrose density gradient ultracentrifugation

The procedure described by Lefkowitz, Williams, Howard and Sigel (1966) was employed for sucrose density gradient fractionation.

Haemagglutination inhibition (HI) test

Standard procedures using guinea-pig erythrocytes were followed. Four haemagglutinating doses of PR8 virus were used in the HI test. One haemagglutinating dose of virus is defined as the amount of virus in the said volume, which produces partial (2^+) agglutination of a 1 per cent suspension of guinea-pig erythrocytes.

Titration of antibody to Rous sarcoma virus.

The methods for *in vivo* tests are described by Sigel, Fugmann and Stolfi (1969) and for *in vitro* tests by Rubin, Cornelius and Fanshier (1961).

RESULTS

TITRATION OF CHICKEN C1

Preliminary microtitrations of C1 in whole chicken serum were performed in the presence of guinea-pig Sup. I in order to determine the optimal ionic strength for this measurement. One drop of dilutions of chicken serum in buffers of varying ionic strength (prepared by mixing appropriate volumes of GVB^{++} and DG^{++}) were reacted (30° for 30 minutes) with one drop of the corresponding buffer and one drop of EAb^{ch} (1×10^8/ml) in the corresponding buffer. One drop of guinea-pig Sup. I diluted in the corresponding buffer, or one drop of buffer alone was then added and haemolysis was allowed to proceed at 37° for 60 minutes. Visual estimation of 50 per cent haemolytic titres (CH^{50}/ml) showed that an ionic strength of 0·075 was optimal for the measurement of chicken C1 (Table 1) under the conditions of test.

TABLE 1

IMMUNE HAEMOLYSIS BY CHICKEN C1 AT VARIOUS IONIC STRENGTHS IN THE PRESENCE AND ABSENCE OF GUINEA-PIG SUP. I

Ionic strength of buffer (I)	Haemolytic titre*	
	Chicken serum	Chicken serum + Guinea-pig Sup. I
0·200	<20	<20
0·150	<20	30
0·075	30	5120
0·050	<20	1280
0·040	<20	960

* Reciprocal of dilution producing approximately 50 per cent haemolysis in microtitre assay.

Although C1 activity was maximal at $I = 0.075$, a rapid loss of activity occurred if diluted chicken serum (or partially purified chicken C1, to be described below) was allowed to stand at this ionic strength before reaction with EAb^{ch}. Inasmuch as a period of standing is required in the fixation phase of a CF test, it was necessary to determine the ionic strength at which chicken C1 would remain stable. It was found that chicken C1 was stable upon standing at $I = 0.15$ for as long as 18–20 hours at 4° and so this ionic strength was used during the fixation phase.

It was also noted that the order of addition of the reagents was critical. Maximal haemolysis with chicken C1 resulted only if it was reacted with EAb^{ch} for at least 30 minutes at 30° before the addition of Sup. I.

Chicken C1 was measured by an endpoint dilution titration incorporating the conditions delineated by the above findings. The data from these titrations were plotted according to the von Krogh transformation (Mayer, 1961) and yielded a straight line

148

between 20 and 80 per cent haemolysis. Titres of chicken Cl obtained from these plots ranged between 8000 and 10,000 CH_{50}/ml.

PREPARATION OF CHICKEN Cl

Chicken Cl could not be isolated from whole serum by precipitation at $I = 0.04$ (pH 7·5), the procedure used to obtain guinea-pig Cl (Nelson, 1961; Nelson *et al.*, 1966), for neither the precipitate nor the supernatant fraction was reactive. Ultimately, it was found that diluting chicken serum 1:8 with 0·02 M acetate buffer, pH 5 (final relative NaCl concentration = 0·02 M, pH 6), resulted in a precipitate containing 60 per cent of the Cl

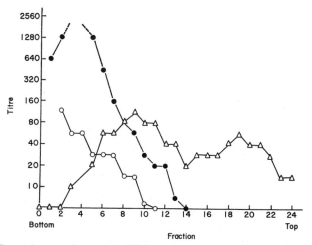

Fig. 1. Sucrose density gradient analysis of Cl activity in whole chicken serum (○) and in a fraction of serum precipitated at 0·02 I, pH 6·0 (●), and of Cl-inhibitory activity in the fraction of chicken serum which was soluble at 0·02 I, pH 6·0 (△).

activity of whole serum. The supernatant fraction was complement-inhibitory. The precipitate was redissolved in ten times the original serum volume of GVB^{++} containing 1 per cent gelatin and was stable upon storage at $-70°$.

SUCROSE DENSITY GRADIENT ULTRACENTRIFUGATION

Whole chicken serum, chicken Cl (precipitated fraction), and the complement-inhibitory supernatant fraction of chicken serum were subjected to sucrose density gradient ultracentrifugation. The sedimentation of chicken Cl (Fig. 1) indicated that, like Cl from guinea-pig (Borsos and Rapp, 1965) and from human (Naff, Pensky and Lepow, 1964) sera, chicken Cl is a macromolecule. The lower reactivity of whole serum in relation to that of partially purified Cl (Fig. 1). suggests the presence of an inhibitor in, or near, the same area.

The ultracentrifuged supernatant fraction was tested for inhibition of chicken Cl (Tamura and Nelson, 1967) and at least two areas of inhibition could be detected (Fig. 1).

Heated chicken antiserum was anticomplementary at dilutions as high as 1:1200. A major portion of this activity could be precipitated from the antiserum along with the Cl by diluting unheated antiserum with water to $I = 0.03$. Antisera treated in this manner were only slightly anticomplementary at dilutions of 1:50 to 1:100 and no antibody activity was lost from the supernatant fraction as measured by haemagglutination inhibition in the PR8 system. All chicken antisera were treated in this manner prior to assay in the Cl-fixation test.

The anticomplementary activity of PR8 virus in allantoic fluid was removed by haemadsorption to guinea-pig erythrocytes at $0°$, centrifugation, and elution at $37°$ into phosphate buffered saline.

Reduction of the anticomplementary activity of RSV-RAV 1 proved to be difficult. Absorption with kaolin, treatment with formalin, heating at $56°$ for up to 60 minutes, as well as purification of the virus by differential centrifugation, washing, sedimentation through 40 per cent sucrose and fractionation on a sucrose density gradient by ultra-centrifugation were equally unsatisfactory for removing the inhibitory action from the virus. However, it was found that reacting the virus with undiluted chicken serum reduced the anticomplementary activity of the virus, and fresh virus destroyed the Cl activity of the serum. Therefore, 3 ml of purified virus were mixed with 3 ml of undiluted chicken serum which was free of RSV-RAV 1 neutralizing antibody and incubated at $30°$ for 30 minutes. Twice in succession, the virus was then pelleted by centrifugation, resuspended in 1 ml of fresh serum and incubated at $30°$ for 30 minutes. The virus was then washed, resuspended in 3 ml of GVB^{++} and tested for inhibition of Cl activity. The inhibitory activity of the virus preparation was reduced from 1:2048 to 1:24 after the three exposures to normal chicken serum. Conversely, the Cl activity of the first sample of serum was reduced in titre from 1:10,000 to 1:12 after exposure to the virus. Virus treated in this manner was then evaluated for use as antigen in Cl-fixation tests.

Cl-FIXATION TESTS

Cl-fixation tests were performed with antigens, chicken antisera and chicken Cl treated or prepared as described above. The detailed method is outlined in Table 2.

1. *PR8 virus and chicken antiserum.* A representative antigen–antibody checkerboard assay with PR8 virus and chicken antiserum to the virus (Table 3) showed that a 1:16 dilution of the virus was optimal for the system and resulted in an antibody titre of between 1:800 and 1:1600. The antiserum was only slightly anticomplementary at dilutions of 1:50 to 1:100.

Sera from a series of bleedings of chickens which had been immunized with the PR8 virus were compared in Cl-fixation and HI activity. On each day sera from approximately 100 chickens were pooled. Each pool was tested on two occasions with identical results. The results, represented in Fig. 2, show that there was good correlation between the two types of test with the exception of the serum from the earliest bleeding (5 days) which showed significantly lower Cl fixation than HI activity. This finding is believed to be a reflection of the predominance of IgM in the 5 day serum.

2. *RSV-RAV 1 and chicken antiserum.* Table 4 shows the results in Cl-fixation with chicken antiserum and two dilutions of RSV-RAV 1 which had been reacted with normal

TABLE 2

METHOD FOR Cl-FIXATION ASSAY

GVB++ (I 0·15)	0·2 ml Antigen
	0·2 ml Cl (5 ClH$_{50}$ units)
	0·2 ml Antibody dilution

18–20 hours at 4°

0·6 ml DG++
(to lower ionic strength to I 0·075)

DGVB++ (I 0·075)	0·2 ml EAb^{ch} (1 × 10^8/ml)
	30 minutes at 30°
	0·2 ml guinea-pig Sup. I (C4,2,3,5,6,7,8,9)
	60 minutes at 37°

Centrifuge and read

TABLE 3

TITRATION OF CHICKEN ANTIBODY TO PR8 VIRUS IN Cl-FIXATION TEST*

Dilution of antigen (PR8 virus)	Antibody dilution (chicken anti-PR8 virus)							
	1/50	1/100	1/200	1/400	1/800	1/1600	1/3200	None
1/8	0	0	0	0	2	3	4	4
1/16	0	0	0	0	0	3	4	4
1/32	0	0	0	0	2	3	4	4
None	2	3	4	4	4	4	4	4

* Cl$_{50}$ units used in test.
0 = no lysis; 4 = complete lysis; 2 = 50 per cent lysis (endpoint).

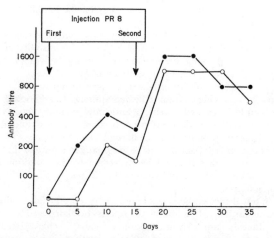

FIG. 2. Cl-fixation (○) and haemagglutination inhibition (●) assays of anti-PR8 virus antibody in chicken sera collected on various days after immunization.

151

chicken serum prior to its utilization as antigen in the test. It may be seen that only the 1:50 dilution of virus was still slightly anticomplementary. An antibody titre of 1:2560 was obtained in the presence of the virus at a 1:100 dilution. This Cl fixation titre correlated well with that of 1:2000 found by *in vitro* and *in vivo* neutralization titrations with the same antiserum.

TABLE 4

TITRATION OF CHICKEN ANTIBODY TO RSV-RAV 1 IN Cl-FIXATION TEST*

Dilutions of antigen (RSV-RAV 1)	Antibody dilutions (chicken anti-RSV-RAV 1)							
	1/80	1/160	1/320	1/640	1/1280	1/2560	1/5120	None
1/50	0	0	0	0	0	0	1	<4
1/100	0	0	0	0	0	2	3	4
None	4	4	4	4	4	4	4	4

* 5 ClH$_{50}$ units used in test.
0 = no lysis; 4 = complete lysis; 2 = 50 per cent lysis (endpoint); <4 = nearly complete lysis.

DISCUSSION

Several factors which have limited the usefulness of a complement fixation test for the measurement of chicken antibodies have been eliminated in the described Cl fixation test. The incompatibility of mammalian Cl and chicken antibody was avoided by using chicken Cl as well as chicken sensitizing antiserum. The use of a guinea-pig serum reagent (Sup. I) containing all of the components of complement except the incompatible Cl increased the sensitivity of measurements of chicken Cl. The use of partially purified Cl avoided any natural antibodies as well as any complement inhibitors present in whole chicken complement.

Other experimental parameters needed to be carefully controlled successfully to employ this method. These included the ionic strength of 0·15 for stability of the chicken Cl during the fixation phase, the ionic strength of 0·075 during the lytic phase, and the reaction of chicken Cl with EAb[ch] prior to the addition of Sup. I.

The marked anticomplementarity of heated chicken serum necessitated the development of a method for removing Cl from unheated antisera. In addition, both the antisera and the antigens had to be treated to remove anticomplementary activity. In this regard the Rous sarcoma virus (RSV-RAV 1) proved of particular interest, and ultimately only a rather tedious absorption procedure using normal chicken serum was successful. The inhibitory effect of this virus did not seem to be enzymatic in nature in that it was heat and formalin resistant and in that it could be overcome by the addition of chicken Cl. Further study is necessary to determine whether this Cl-inactivating activity is an intrinsic property of the virion itself.

The Cl-fixation test described here was found to be reproducible and sensitive for the detection of chicken antibody. In addition, the results correlated well with those of certain other methods ordinarily employed to measure antibodies in chicken serum. Owing to its complexity, this test may not be the one of choice when other, simpler means are available. However, when the alternative is an expensive and time-consuming method, this test should prove of particular value. Once the reagents have been prepared, it offers a relatively fast and simple procedure for the routine measurement of complement fixing antibodies of chicken serum.

ACKNOWLEDGMENTS

We thank Miss Eva K. Hultqvist and Mr Edward J. Rooks for skilful technical assistance. The work was supported by Contract No. PH43–67–1187 within the Special Virus Leukaemia Program of the National Cancer Institute, National Institution of Health, Public Health Service.

REFERENCES

BENSON, H. N., BRUMFIELD, H. P. and POMEROY, B. S. (1961). 'Requirement of avian C'1 for fixation of guinea pig complement by avian antibody–antigen complexes.' *J. Immunol.*, **87**, 616.

BORSOS, T. and RAPP, H. J. (1965). 'Estimation of molecular size of complement components by sephadex chromatography.' *J. Immunol.*, **94**, 510.

BRUMFIELD, H. P., BENSON, H. N. and POMEROY, B. S. (1961). 'Procedure for modified complement fixation test with turkey, duck, and chicken serum antibody.' *Avian Dis.*, **5**, 270.

LEFKOWITZ, S. S., WILLIAMS, J. A., HOWARD, B. E. and SIGEL, M. M. (1966). 'Adenovirus antibody measured by the passive hemagglutination test.' *J. Bact.*, **91**, 205.

MAYER, M. M. (1961). *Experimental Immunochemistry* (Ed. by E. A. Kabat and M. M. Mayer). Charles C. Thomas, Springfield, Illinois.

NAFF, G. B., PENSKY, J. and LEPOW, I. H. (1964). 'The macromolecular nature of the first component of human complement.' *J. exp. Med.*, **119**, 593.

NELSON, R. A. (1961). 'Mechanisms of cell and tissue damage produced by immune reactions.' *2nd International Symposium on Immunopathology* (Ed. by P. Grabar and P. Miescher), p. 819. Schwabe, Basel.

NELSON, R. A., JENSEN, J. J., GIGLI, I. and TAMURA. N. (1966). 'Methods for the separation, purification and measurement of nine components of hemolytic complement in guinea-pig serum.' *Immunochemistry*, **3**, 111.

OKAZAKI, W., PURCHASE, H. G., FREDRICKSON, T. N. and BURMESTER, B. B. (1962). 'Modification of complement fixation test for estimation of Rous sarcoma virus antibodies in turkey and chicken serums.' *Proc. Soc. exp. Biol. (N.Y.)*, **111**, 377.

ORLANS, E., ROSE, M. E. and CLAPP, K. H. (1962). 'Fowl antibody. V. The interactions of fresh and heated fowl serum and of guinea-pig complement measured by the lysis of sensitized red cells.' *Immunology*, **5**, 649.

RICE, C. E. (1947). 'Atypical behaviour of certain avian antisera in complement fixation tests.' *Canad. J. comp. Med.*, **11**, 236.

ROSE, M. E. and ORLANS, E. (1962a). 'Fowl antibody. III. Its haemolytic activity with complements of various species and some properties of fowl complement.' *Immunology*, **5**, 633.

ROSE, M. E. and ORLANS, E. (1962b). 'Fowl antibody. IV. The estimation of haemolytic fowl complement.' *Immunology*, **5**, 642.

SIGEL, M. M., FUGMANN, R. A. and STOLFI, R. L. (1970). 'Immunity and Tolerance in Oncogenesis.' *IVth Int. Conf. on Cancer. Perugia.* (Ed. by L. Severi), p. 117. Div. of Cancer Res., Univ. of Perugia.

RUBIN, H., CORRELIUS, A. and FAUSHIER, L. (1961). 'The pattern of congenital transmission of an avian leukosis virus.' *Proc. nat. Acad. Sci. (Wash.)*, **47**, 1058.

TAMURA, N. and NELSON, R. A. (1967). 'Three naturally-occurring inhibitors of components of complements in guinea pig and rabbit serum.' *J. Immunol.*, **99**, 582.

A Transient Cytotoxic Host Response to the Rous Sarcoma Virus–Induced Transplantation Antigen (34851)

CLIFFORD J. BELLONE AND MORRIS POLLARD

Tumor-specific transplantation antigens (TSTA) were demonstrated in chemically induced neoplasms by Foley (1) and by Prehn and Main (2). Subsequently, TSTA were reported in other experimental tumor systems, *i.e.*, in "spontaneous" tumors, and in tumors induced by oncogenic viruses, chemical carcinogens, and by implanted inert materials. Current data indicated that the immunity engendered by the host against the TSTA involves mechanisms similar to those which are responsible for homograft rejection. Many hypotheses have been postulated to explain the growth of tumors as regards host responses to homografts. Some involve the antibody enhancement phenomena (3) immunodepression in the case of chemically induced tumors (4), and tolerance or paralysis (5). Mikulska *et al.* (6), have demonstrated a suppressed immunological status in the host to its tumor, which recovers after removal of the tumor. This suggests that the host is capable of initiating an immune response, but in the process of tumor growth the immune mechanism is "turned off" or "paralyzed." The information reported here attempts to examine the time-relationship of this phenomenon after implantation of tumor cells. It involves *in vitro* cell culture techniques by which the cell-associated immunological status of the host can be assessed.

Materials and Methods. A transplantable fibrosarcoma was induced in newborn female

[1] This work was supported by the John A. Hartford Foundation, the U.S. Public Health Service, and Allen County Cancer Society, Indiana.

inbred Fischer rats by subcutaneous inoculation of 10^4 PFU of Schmidt-Ruppin strain Rous sarcoma virus. The virus was obtained from Dr. Ray Bryan, National Cancer Institute, Bethesda, Maryland. A selected primary solid tumor, which appeared approximately $4\frac{1}{2}$ months later, was excised and minced under asceptic conditions. The small fragments, in minimal essential media (MEM), were then aspirated vigorously in a 1-ml syringe and 0.1 ml of this cell suspension was then inoculated subcutaneously into the interscapular region of newborn Fischer rats. The tumor was transplanted twice through newborn rats and thereafter into rats of weanling age. Tumors of the fourth to the sixth cell passages in inbred weanling female Fischer rats were used in the experiments which are described below. Four to ten animals were used to assess immunity for each interval studied. However, at times lymphoid cells from two different animals were pooled.

In order to assess the cell-mediated immune status of the host, the passaged tumor was excised aseptically into Eagle's MEM at pH 7. The tumor tissue was then minced with scissors to very fine fragments, and washed once in MEM; and the tissue fragments were then resuspended in prewarmed 0.25% solution of trypsin (Difco 1:250) in phosphate-buffered saline (PBS) for 30 min at 37° in a combination water bath–shaker. The dispersed cells were then decanted through sterile gauze, centrifuged, and washed twice in MEM at 4°. The cells were counted by hemocytometer and 10^6 morphologically intact cells (88% viable as determined by trypan blue exclusion test) were inoculated subcutaneously in the dorsal region of the rat.

TABLE I. Response of Lymphoid Cells from RSV Tumor-Bearing Rats Inoculated with 10^6 Tumor Cells.

Days after inoculation of RSV tumor cells	RSV tumor cells (% survival ± SE)		
	Lymphoid cells from:		
	Normal rats		Tumor-bearing rats
10	100 ± 16.9	(4)[a]	90.5 ± 8.26
15–21	100 ± 4.9	(9)	47.3 ± 6.8
22–29	100 ± 8.9	(11)	102 ± 5.56
32–38	100 ± 3.8	(10)	126 ±16

[a] Number of rats in each group.

Assays for host sensitization to the inoculated tumor cells were performed by *in vitro* cytotoxicity tests (7). RSV tumor cells, propagated in tissue culture, were suspended in Waymouth's 752/1 medium (Gibco) plus 10% heat-inactivated calf serum; and 3×10^5 and 1×10^6 cells were seeded in Leighton tubes and in 25-mm petri dishes, respectively. Twenty-four hours later the inoculated and uninoculated control animals were anesthetized by ether, exsanguinated from the heart, and the brachial, inguinal, and mesenteric lymph nodes were removed aseptically, pooled, and washed in MEM. The lymph nodes were teased through a sterile 60-mesh stainless steel screen, the cells were washed twice and adjusted to a final concentration of 1 and 1.5–2.0×10^6 cells per ml in Waymouth's medium containing 5% heat-inactivated fetal calf serum. 2×10^6 of the lymph node cells were added to the Leighton tubes and 4.5–6.0 million cells were added to each petri dish of "target" tumor cells. The mixed cultures were incubated for 48 hr at 37° in a mixture of 5% CO_2 and 95% air and then examined for surviving target tumor cells. The nutrient medium was replaced by PBS, and then by 2 ml of 0.25% trypsin. After incubation at 37° for 20–25 min, chilled PBS was added to the cell–trypsin mixture. The detached cells were then counted by hemocytometer and from this the percentages of surviving tumor cells were calculated. Tumor cells and lymphocytes were differentiated on the basis of size and morphology.

Results. The data in Table I indicate that lymphocytes from the rats which had been inoculated 10 days previously with 10^6 viable tumor cells showed a low-level cytotoxic response. The maximum response which was reflected in the survival of only 51.1% of the tumor cells was observed on Days 15–21 after the inoculation of tumor cells. From Days 22 on the lymphoid cells from the tumor-bearing rats did not destroy the target cells. Tumors appeared in the inoculated rats at 8–10 days after inoculation of tumor cells. No exact correlation was found between tumor size and the immune status of the host; however, average tumor size of approximately 2-cm diameter coincided with maximum cytotoxic response. Average tumor diameter in the nonresponsive rats was approximately 5 cm.

The data in Table II portray a similar pattern of transient response, but the time sequence of the cytotoxic effect appeared earlier. These rats were inoculated with the same line of tumor cells, but after it had been passaged four times in tissue culture. Inoculation of 10^6 tumor cells (96% viable by trypan blue exclusion test) induced palpable tumors 7 days after inoculation as compared with 8–10 days in the previous experiments. The accelerated appearance of tumors may be a result of a higher percentage of viable cells in the inoculum and/or of some selective enhancement of the tumor cells through their propagation in tissue culture.

Specificity of the cell-associated immune reaction is demonstrated in Table II. Lymphoid cells which destroyed RSV tumor cells were inactive on sarcoma cells which had been induced in Fischer rats by polyoma virus.

Discussion. The experimental data recorded here support the recent report of Barski and Youn (8) on a transient host-immune response to inoculated Rauscher virus-transformed T5 tumor cells, with a subsequent state of "paralysis." Our data suggest that an actively growing solid tumor in some way "paralyzes" or reverses the initial cell-mediated immune responses of the host, as determined by *in vitro* cytotoxicity tests (6, 8). This is supported by experimentally derived results involving X-ray-inactivated tu-

Days after tu-mor inoculation	RSV tumor cells (% survival ± SE)		Polyoma tumor cells (% survival ± SE)	
	Lymphoid cells from:		Lymphoid cells from:	
	Normal rats	Tumor-bearing rats	Normal rats	Tumor-bearing rats
9	100 ± 3.0	51.6 ± 6.2	100 ± 16.7	117 ± 20.9
16	100 ± 13.4	114.9 ± 7.14	—	—

mor cells, and by surgical extirpation of tumor after which the lymphoid tissue of the host then regained the capacity for a cytotoxic response through appropiate *in vitro* tests (6, 8). While our results do not clarify the mechanism(s) involved in this state of "paralysis," antibody enhancement, tolerance, or some humoral immune-depressive factor (9) associated with a population of growing tumor cells have been offered as possible explanations (10). Possibly, one or more of these factors are operating to cause the unresponsive state of the lymphoid cells on the target tissue. This observed phenomenon has been explained by the fact that the majority of sensitized lymphoid cells are assembled at tumor site. However, from histological examinations of germ-free tumors significant numbers of lymphoid cells have not been observed in or around the tumors.

Our data suggested that there was an "enhancing" effect of the "paralyzed" lymphoid cells on the target tissue. Although this may not be significant statistically, there is nevertheless a suggestive trend toward a stimulatory effect in excess of the normal "feeder" effect associated with exposure to unsensitized lymphoid cells.

If tumor cells continue to grow in the host as a result of immunological disability, then control will depend on some means of immunological enhancement. Possibly, tumor cells are more efficient as immunological depressants than "normal" tissues, and it could be important to determine its nature. It is significant that tumor-bearing rats whose lymphoid cells had reached the "paralyzed," or nonresponsive stage, *in vitro*, were physically indistinguishable from tumor-free con-

trols when judged by size, by physical condition, and by general appearance. Thus, the lack of cytoxic cell response in the *in vitro* tests could not be attributed to a general state of debilitation in the tumor-bearing hosts.

Recently some evidence has accumulated in our laboratory that the RSV TSTA may have been altered, decreased quantitatively, or lost entirely. Preliminary data have shown that when the same RSV tumor that was used throughout all of the above experiments was used after 16 passages in Fischer rats no reactions were found when assayed during the usual time intervals. This has also been the case with another RSV primary now in the 5th animal passage. There are reports in the literature where TSTA in solid tumors, induced by so-called defective oncogenic viruses, appeared to have been lost (11). Further work on this problem is currently being conducted in our laboratory. It may be important, in this regard, to limit such experiments to "primary" tumors or to close derivatives thereof.

Summary. This report is concerned with the time-relationship of cell-mediated immune reactions by hosts with expanding transplanted solid tumors. Inoculation of 10^6 serially passaged tumor cells elicited peak lymphocyte cytotoxic responses between 16 and 21 days followed by a state of immunological "paralysis." Rats which were inoculated with 10^6 tumor cells which had been passaged four additional times in tissue culture gave lymphocytes with peak cytotoxic effects at 9 days after implantation and "paralysis" by 16 days. A stimulatory effect over and above the normal "feeder" effect by unsensitized lymphoid cells was noted when "paralyzed" cells were overlayed on the target cells. This "paralysis" could not be attributed to a general state of debilitation in the tumor-bearing hosts.

1. Foley, E. J., Cancer Res. 13, 835 (1953).
2. Prehn, R. T., and Main, J. M., J. Nat. Cancer Inst. 18, 769 (1957).
3. Hellstrom, I., Hellstrom, K. E., Evans, C. A., Heppner, G. H., Pierce, G. E., and Yang, J. P. S., Proc. Nat. Acad. Sci. U.S.A. 62, 362 (1969).
4. Stjernsward, J., J. Nat. Cancer Inst. 40, 13 (1968).
5. Klein, E., and Klein, G., Cancer Res. 25, 851 (1965).
6. Mikulska, Z. B., Smith, C., and Alexander, P., J. Nat. Cancer Inst. 36, 29 (1966).
7. Rosenau, W., in "Cell-Bound Antibodies" (B. Amos and H. Koprowski, eds.), p. 75. Wistar Institute Press, Philadelphia, Pennsylvania (1963).
8. Barski, G., and Youn, J. K., J. Nat. Cancer Inst. 43, 111 (1969).
9. Mowbray, J. F., Transplantation 1, 15 (1963).
10. Zacharia, T. P., Doctoral Thesis, University of Notre Dame, Notre Dame, Indiana (1968).
11. Deichman, G. I., and Kluchareva, T. E., J. Nat. Cancer Inst. 36, 647 (1966).

The Presence of Avian Leukosis Virus Group-Specific Antibodies in Chicken Sera[1]

FRIEDA K. ROTH, PAUL MEYERS, AND ROBERT M. DOUGHERTY

INTRODUCTION

The antigens of the avian leukosis-sarcoma viruses can be classified into two groups: (1) type-specific (ts) antigens which react with virus-neutralizing antibodies and are components of the viral envelope (Ishizaki and Vogt, 1966) and (2) group-specific (gs) antigens which do not react with neutralizing antibodies and are considered to be internal components of all viruses of the group (Huebner et al., 1963, 1964; Bauer and Schäfer, 1965, 1966; Payne et al., 1966; Kelloff and Vogt, 1966).

The gs antigens are capable of inducing complement-fixing (CF), immunofluorescing, and precipitating antibodies in the sera of hamsters bearing tumors induced by Rous sarcoma viruses (RSV) (Huebner et al., 1963; Kelloff and Vogt, 1966; Berman and Sarma, 1965; Bauer and Janda, 1967; Allen, 1967; Armstrong, 1969; Roth and Dougherty, 1969). These antigens can also be detected with the sera of rabbits immunized with disrupted avian myeloblastosis virus (Eckert et al., 1964a, b; Bauer and Schäfer, 1966).

Direct CF tests to examine chicken sera for gs antibodies cannot be performed as chicken antisera do not fix guinea pig complement (Rice, 1948). Kelloff and Vogt (1966) were unable to detect these antibodies in chicken antisera with the fluorescent antibody technique. This failure to demonstrate gs antibodies in infected chickens (the natural host) had an apparently logical explanation. Chicken embryos, otherwise free of infectious ALV, often contained ALV gs antigen (Dougherty and DiStefano, 1966;

[1] This investigation was supported by U. S. Public Health Service Research Grant No. CA10148 from the National Cancer Institute.

158

TABLE 1

TABLE 1
STRAINS OF VIRUS USED

Virus	Antigenic subgroup[a]	Source
RSV strains		
Schmidt-Ruppin[b]	B	C. G. Ahlström
Prague[b]	C	J. Svoboda
ALV strains		
RAV-1 (Bryan RAV)[c]	A	R. M. Dougherty
RAV-6 (Harris RAV)[d]	B	R. M. Dougherty
ALV-F42	A	P. Biggs
RSV Pseudotypes		
B-RSV (RAV-1)[e]	A	R. M. Dougherty
B-RSV (RAV-6)[e]	B	R. M. Dougherty

[a] Duff and Vogt (1969); Ishizaki and Vogt (1966).
[b] Cloned by repeated single-focus isolation.
[c] Isolated from Bryan RSV by end point dilution method (Rubin and Vogt, 1962).
[d] Isolated from Harris RSV by end point dilution method (Rubin and Vogt, 1962).
[e] Produced by superinfection of "NP" cells (Hanafusa et al., 1963).

Dougherty et al., 1967). The distribution of this antigen in crosses of two inbred lines of chickens resembled that of a genetically inherited trait controlled by a dominant autosomal gene (Payne and Chubb, 1968). It was postulated (Payne and Chubb, 1968) that the antigen represented phenotypic expression of viral genes that had become integrated with the host genome. Presence of gs antigen in embryos was thought to induce immune tolerance which explained absence of gs antibodies in response to ALV infection. There was also evidence that mice and cats were tolerant to their homologous gs leukemia virus antigen (Geering et al., 1966; Huebner and Todaro, 1969).

This concept was challenged by the findings of Armstrong (1969), who detected ALV gs antibodies in chicken antisera by immunodiffusion tests. Recently Rabotti and Blackham (1970), using a complement-fixation inhibition (CFI) test, revealed gs antibodies in the sera of fowls immunized with RSV. The present report supports these findings. Antibodies were found by CFI tests in sera from chickens immunized with two strains of ALV but were not found in chickens congenitally infected with ALV and immunized with the same or heterologous virus strains.

MATERIALS AND METHODS

Viruses. The strains of RSV and ALV used are characterized in Table 1. The virus stocks were supernatant tissue culture fluids from infected cell cultures and were prepared in this laboratory. All viruses were stored frozen at either $-65°$ or $-78°$.

Neutralizing antibody assays. For quantitation of neutralizing antibody content of the chicken sera, the log of the serum dilution that neutralized 50% of the virus (log ND_{50}) was calculated (Dulbecco et al., 1956; Dougherty et al., 1960; Meyers and Dougherty, 1971).

Sources of chickens and fertile eggs. Leukosis-free: Fertile White Leghorn eggs from a specific pathogen free flock were obtained from SPAFAS, Incorporated, Norwich, Connecticut. This flock is largely free of intercurrent ALV infection and was therefore used as a source of eggs for ALV-free control animals as well as for the production of artificially congenitally infected birds.

Congenitally infected: A flock of chickens congenitally infected with a subgroup A strain of leukosis virus, ALV-F42, and maintained in this laboratory (DiStefano and Dougherty, 1966) was used as the source of some chickens. Artificially congenitally infected chickens, produced by injecting SPAFAS embryos with ALV-F42, were also used (Meyers and Dougherty, 1971).

Preparation of antigens. Group-specific antigens were made from chick embryo fibroblast tissue cultures infected with either the Schmidt-Ruppin (SR) or Prague (Pr) strains of RSV or from Rous-associated virus

159

(RAV-1). Details regarding the antigenic preparations have been published elsewhere (Roth and Dougherty, 1969).

Preparation of antisera. In order to determine the antibody responses of uninfected control birds and congenitally infected birds to RAV-1 and RAV-6, animals of various ages were injected with virus and bled at intervals. Details have been previously described (Meyers and Dougherty, 1971). The sera were heated at 56° for 30 min prior to use in neutralization or CFI tests.

CFI tests. Chicken serum does not fix guinea pig complement in the usual system. The inhibition test is based on the fact that chicken serum combines with the antigen and blocks its combining sites (Rice, 1948). Thus mammalian antibody (which does fix complement) is prevented from reacting with the antigen, and complement-fixation is blocked. In addition to antigen, chicken serum, complement and the hemolytic system, mammalian antibody directed to the test antigen is used. The mammalian antibody used in our tests was ALV gs antiserum from hamsters with sarcomas induced by SR-RSV. Sera collected from hamsters bearing large primary tumors were heated at 56° for 30 min (Roth and Dougherty, 1969). Several positive hamster sera were pooled. This serum pool had a titer of 1:300 against 4 units of SR-RSV gs antigen prepared from infected chick embryo fibroblast tissue cultures.

The preparation of gs antigen used in the CFI tests was from Pr-RSV-infected chicken cell cultures and had a direct CF titer of approximately 1:4000. It was necessary to standardize this antigen for each run. For preliminary standardization, the highest dilution of antigen was determined that give a 50% lytic reaction in our standard (Roth and Dougherty, 1969) CF test using 5 C′H$_{50}$ units of complement, and a 1:75 dilution (4 units) of the RSV-immune hamster serum pool. This antigen dilution was considered as 1 unit. For the CFI test, 4 units of antigen were incubated with 2-fold dilutions of chicken antisera at 37° for 2 hr. All the wells then received the hamster immune serum (dilution 1:75) and 5 units of guinea pig complement. After the plates were incubated overnight at 4°, the indicator system was added. The titer of the test was expressed as the reciprocal of the highest dilution of chicken serum capable of binding the antigen and inhibiting complement fixation by the hamster serum (the highest dilution of chicken serum in which 50% hemolysis occurred).

Purification of chicken immunoglobulins. Salt fractionation of chicken sera was carried out as described by Benedict (1967). After the sera were centrifuged at 700 rpm for 10 min at 4°, the following operations were performed on the clarified sera at room temperature. Globulins were precipitated by the slow addition to the serum of Na$_2$SO$_4$ to a final concentration of 0.18 g/ml. After standing for 30 min, the precipitate was recovered by centrifugation at 200 g for 15 min and redissolved in 0.1 M Tris-HCl buffer in 1.0 M NaCl, pH 8.0, to the original serum volume. Two further precipitations were made by adding Na$_2$SO$_4$ to a final concentration of 0.14 g/ml. After the final precipitation, the globulins were redissolved and dialyzed against the Tris buffer for 48 hr at 4°. After dialysis the preparation was cleared by centrifugation at 200 g for 20 min, the volume measured and a sample taken for assay of antibody activity.

The salt-precipitated globulin preparation was applied to a column of Sephadex G-200 to effect the separation of IgM and IgG (Flodin and Killander, 1962). A 2.5 × 100 cm Pharmacia column, with a bed volume of approximately 485 ml and a void volume of approximately 150 ml (as determined by elution of Blue Dextran 200) was employed. Elution with 0.1 ml Tris-HCl buffer in 1.0 M NaCl took place at 4°, and 8-ml fractions were collected. Protein concentration of the elutant was determined by absorption at 280 nm on a Zeiss spectrophotometer. Pools made of the peak protein fractions were concentrated by ultrafiltration in a Diaflo apparatus (Amicon Corp., Lexington, Massachusetts) utilizing an XM-100 A membrane. After concentration to a volume of approximately 5 ml, samples were taken and the pools were recycled on Sephadex G-200 as before to obtain single protein peaks. These peak fractions were again pooled, concentrated to approximately 5 ml and assayed for antibody activity.

TABLE 2
Complement-Fixation Inhibition Box Titration

Pr-RSV gs antigen	Chicken antiserum dilution[a]							
Units	2	4	8	16	32	64	128	256
8	4[b]	4	4	4	2	0	0	0
4	4	4	4	4	4	2	0	0
2	4	4	4	4	4	4	4	4

[a] Reciprocal of dilution.
[b] Hemolysis, reading scale of 0–4.

RESULTS

Demonstration, by CFI Tests, of gs Antibodies in Sera of Chickens Injected with RAV-6

Table 2 shows a representative reaction, in the CFI test, of a chicken immune serum against 8, 4, and 2 units of gs antigen prepared from CEF infected with Pr-RSV. The chicken gs antibody titer was 32 with 8 antigen units, 64 with 4 antigen units, and >256 with 2 antigen units.

In order to demonstrate the group-specificity of this test, 8 antisera from control birds that had been injected with RAV-6 (ALV subgroup B) at 6 weeks of age and bled at 15 weeks were tested with 4 units each of gs antigen prepared from CEF infected with RAV-1 (subgroup A), SR-RSV (subgroup B), or Pr-RSV (subgroup C). The data in Table 3 show that the titers obtained with each individual antiserum are similar with the three different gs antigen preparations, and provides evidence that the CFI test is detecting gs antigen.

Responses of Control and Congenitally Infected Birds to RAV-1

The experiments were originally set up to study chicken ts antibody responses (Meyers and Dougherty, 1971). Uninfected control birds and congenitally infected birds of various ages were injected with RAV-1, an ALV of subgroup A, bled at intervals and the presence of ts antibodies ascertained. Uninfected birds received one intravenous injection of 1.0 ml of RAV-1 containing 10^7 infectious units/ml. Congenitally infected birds received two intraperitoneal injections of 1.0 ml of the same virus in Freund's com-

TABLE 3
Group-Specificity of the Complement-Fixation Inhibition Test

Chicken serum No.	CFI titer[a] of chicken anti-RAV-6-sera with 4 units of gs antigen prepared from CEF infected with		
	RAV-1, subgroup A	SR-RSV, subgroup B	Pr-RSV, subgroup C
1766	4	4	8
1769	64	64	128
1772	2	4	2
1773	16	32	32
1778	2	4	2
1779	8	16	16
1781	8	16	16
1783	2	2	4

[a] Reciprocal of chicken serum dilution.

plete adjuvant (1:1, v/v) on days 1 and 3. Control and congenitally infected birds of ages 2½, 6, and 23 weeks were utilized in order to give a range of ages representing early, intermediate and adult levels of immunocompetence. All control birds were purchased from SPAFAS, Inc. The 6-week and 23-week congenitally infected birds were from the flock maintained by this laboratory, while the 2½ week congenitally infected birds were hatched and reared from SPAFAS eggs that had been injected with ALV-F42 as 7-day embryos.

The ts antibody response was measured by neutralization of the homologous sarcoma virus pseudotype B-RSV (RAV-1). Attempts to break tolerance to the ALV-F42 (subgroup A) congenitally infected birds were unsuccessful with the exception of one bird (Meyers and Dougherty, 1971).

After publication of the paper by Rabotti and Blackham (1970), these chicken sera which had been kept at −20°, were examined for gs antibodies by means of the CFI test. The gs antibody responses of these birds are presented in Table 4. Although the number of birds used in each age group was small, certain trends appeared. The congenitally infected birds of all ages failed to produce gs antibodies. Low-titer gs antibodies to RAV-1 first appeared in the 2½-week control group at 5 weeks after challenge and in the 6-week control group at 8 weeks after challenge. There was a complete lack of gs

161

TABLE 4

gs ANTIBODY RESPONSES OF CONTROL AND CONGENITALLY INFECTED CHICKENS TO RAV-1
INJECTED AT VARIOUS AGES

Group	Age at injection with RAV-1 (weeks)	Number with antibody over total at time (weeks)			Average CFI titer[a] of birds with antibody
		2	5	8	
Control	2½	0/8	1/10	3/7	4
	6	0/7	0/8	1/4	4
	23	0/5	0/5	0/2	—
Congenitally infected (ALV-F42)	2½	0/6	0/9	0/3	—
	6	0/9	0/10	0/3	—
	23	ND[b]	0/1	0/1	—

[a] Titer expressed as reciprocal of chicken serum dilution.
[b] Not done.

antibody response in the birds injected at 23 weeks of age within the 8-week test period.

Responses of Control and Congenitally Infected Birds to RAV-6

Further tests of ts antibody response were made by injecting chickens congenitally infected with ALV-F42 and control birds of various ages with RAV-6, which is a member of subgroup B and antigenically unrelated to ALV-F42 or RAV-1 in terms of the envelope antigens (Meyers and Dougherty, 1971). Control and congenitally infected birds were injected either intravenously with a single 1.0 ml dose of RAV-6 containing 10^5 infectious units/ml or intraperitoneally with two 1.0-ml doses of the same virus preparation in Freund's complete adjuvant (1:1, v/v) on days 0 and 3. The ts antibody response, measured by neutralization of the homologous sarcoma virus pseudotype B-RSV (RAV-6), was determined at various time intervals after injection. Meyers and Dougherty (1971) found that the ts antibody response to a subgroup B ALV challenge in the subgroup A ALV congenitally infected birds was age-dependent. Although there seemed to be no impairment in birds challenged at 25 weeks, the congenitally infected birds injected with RAV-6 at 6 weeks showed a marked depression in ts antibody response to this virus. In the 2½-week-old group only 8% of the congenitally infected birds responded.

These chicken sera, used for the neutralization tests, were stored at −20°. Many were examined for gs antibodies by means of the CFI test. Not all the individual sera were available, as some had been used up in the previous ts antibody tests. Table 5 shows the gs antibody responses of the control and congenitally infected birds. In the control group of birds injected at 25 weeks of age, 1/3 birds tested at 8 weeks responded with antibody and at 12–20 weeks, 0/9 responded. It was unfortunate that a later blood sample from the positive bird was unavailable. In the congenitally infected group injected at 25 weeks there was no response at all within the test period.

The data presented in Table 5 indicate that control birds injected at 6 weeks elicited a greater gs antibody response than chickens injected at 25 weeks. Bleedings at 8 weeks showed that 8/9 birds responded, and bleedings at 12–20 weeks showed that 12/19 birds had gs antibodies. Although more birds responded after intraperitoneal injections with Freund's adjuvant, higher antibody titers were obtained in those birds which had received intravenous injections. The differences in titer may not be significant. It will be noted that one bird had gs antibodies as early as 5–6 weeks after injection. In the congenitally infected group injected at 6 weeks there was no gs antibody response at all within the test period.

The results of the same experiment performed on birds 2½ weeks old are also shown in Table 5: 58% of the birds responded at the 5–6 week bleeding, 71% responded at the 8 week bleeding, and 68% had antibodies at the 12–20 week bleeding. More birds responded after intraperitoneal

TABLE 5

gs Antibody Responses in Congenitally Infected and Control Chickens Injected at Various Ages with RAV-6

Group	Age at injection with RAV-6 (weeks)	Route of injection	Number with gs antibody over total at time (weeks)			Average CFI titer[a] of birds with antibody
			5–6	8	12–20	
Control	2½	I.V.	4/9	2/5	5/9	14
		I.P.	7/10	8/9	8/10	24
		Total	11/19 (58%)	10/14 (71%)	13/19 (68%)	19
	6	I.V.	0/1	8/9	5/9	36
		I.P.	1/1	ND[b]	7/10	6
		Total	1/2 (50%)	—	12/19 (63%)	21
	25	I.V.	ND	1/2	0/5	8
		I.P.	ND	0/1	0/4	—
		Total	ND	1/3 (33%)	0/9 (0%)	
Congenitally infected (ALV-F42)	2½	I.V.	0/3	0/4	0/4	—
		I.P.	0/6	0/7	0/7	—
		Total	0/9	0/11	0/11	
	6	I.V.	0/4	0/5	0/6	—
		I.P.	0/1	0/2	0/4	—
		Total	0/5	0/7	0/10	
	25	I.V.	0/1	0/1	0/6	—
		I.P.	ND	ND	0/4	—
		Total	—	—	0/10	

[a] Titer expressed as reciprocal of chicken serum dilution.
[b] Not done.

injections with Freund's adjuvant and their sera had greater antibody titers than the sera from intravenously injected chickens. In the congenitally infected group injected at 2½ weeks, no birds made gs antibodies within the test period.

Comparison of Ts and Gs Antibody Titers

A total of 70 sera from control chickens (i.e., not congenitally infected) injected at various ages with either RAV-1 or RAV-6 were examined for both neutralizing and gs antibodies. There was no significant difference in antibody response to the two viruses. In Table 6 is a comparison of log ND_{50} values with percentage of sera positive for gs antibodies. The greatest number of gs positive sera were those having log ND_{50} values of 3.1–>4, and the most potent sera had log ND_{50} values of 3.1–4. All the gs-positive sera had values >2.3. It was surprising that the sera with the greatest neutralizing activity (log ND_{50} values >4) did not have the greatest gs antibody titers. In many instances sera with high neutralizing activity did not contain any gs antibodies detectable by the CFI test. The titers of gs antibodies in the chicken antisera ranged from 2 to 128.

Of 31 ALV-F42 congenitally infected birds of various ages injected with RAV-6 and bled at 16–20 weeks, 12, or approximately 40%, had neutralizing activity (log ND_{50} values ranging from 2.0 to 3.9) in their sera. However, none of these twelve sera contained gs antibodies.

Fractionation of Chicken Serum Antibodies

Fractionation of 2 chicken sera which contained gs antibodies was carried out to determine which classes of immunoglobulins were involved in the antibody response. Five milli-

TABLE 6

Comparison of ts and gs Antibody Activity in Antisera from Control Chickens Injected Either with RAV-1 or RAV-6

log ND_{50}	Number with gs antibody over total number of birds	% with gs antibody	Average titer[a] of gs antibody
<1.0-2	0/8	0	—
2.1-3	4/15	27	24.5
3.1-4	22/29	76	38.1
>4	13/18	72	11.9
Total	39/70	56	

[a] Titer is expressed as reciprocal of the dilution of chicken serum.

TABLE 7

Fractionation of Chicken Antibody

Fraction	Parameter	Serum numbers	
		1449	2571
Original	log ND_{50}	4.6	ND^b
serum	CFI titer[a]	64	128
Na_2SO_4-	log ND_{50}	4.1	ND
precipitated globulins	CFI titer	32	AC^c
First IgM	log ND_{50}	1.5	ND
	CFI titer	<4	AC
Recycled	log ND_{50}	1.3	ND
IgM	CFI titer	<8	<8
First IgG	log ND_{50}	3.6	ND
	CFI titer	32	ND
Recycled	log ND_{50}	3.7	ND
IgG	CFI titer	64	64

[a] Titer is expressed as the reciprocal of the chicken serum dilution.

[b] Not done.

[c] Anticomplementary.

liters of each serum was used as the starting material. Globulins were precipitated by Na_2SO_4 and applied to a column of Sephadex G-200 to effect the separation of IgM and IgG. The IgM and IgG fractions were recycled and concentrated to approximately 5 ml of each. CFI tests were performed on samples taken at each step of the procedure and neutralization tests were done on all samples of one of the sera (1449). These data

are presented in Table 7. In both sera the gs antibody activity was present in the IgG fractions and was not present in the IgM fractions. Our finding that the neutralizing antibody was also present in the IgG fraction agrees with that of Meyers (1970) who fractionated 14 antisera to ALV subgroup A or B viruses and found that most of the neutralizing antibody was associated with the IgG fraction.

DISCUSSION

Three lines of evidence confirm that the CFI test used in these studies detected chicken antibodies to ALV gs antigen. First, as shown in Table 3, chicken antisera reacted equally with gs antigens of viruses representing 3 distinct envelope serotypes of avian leukosis-sarcoma viruses. Second, the specificity of the CFI test is determined by the most specific component of the antigen–antibody reaction used in the direct part of the test, in this case hamster antiserum against SR-RSV-induced hamster sarcoma. The evidence is clear that this reagent contains ALV gs antibodies, but no antibodies against type-specific antigens (Huebner et al., 1963, 1964). Finally, chickens congenitally infected with ALV of one subgroup failed to make CFI antibodies when challenged with ALV of a different subgroup. Thus, immune tolerance in chickens to gs antigen, as detected by CFI, is group-specific.

These results confirm reports that chickens make antibodies to ALV gs antigen that can be detected by immunodiffusion (Armstrong, 1969) or CFI (Rabotti and Blackham, 1970). Such antibodies are also detectable with the paired radioiodine-labeled antibody technique (Yohn et al., 1971). Our results show that gs antibodies develop later than neutralizing antibodies (Meyers, 1970) and most CFI titers are not high. This may explain why Kelloff and Vogt (1966) were unable to detect gs activity in chicken antisera to a number of strains of ALV or RSV using fluorescent antibodies. These authors were cautious in interpreting their results and suggested that the method might not be sensitive enough to detect small amounts of gs antibody. Others were less inhibited in drawing conclusions from these data.

Dougherty and DiStefano (1966) showed that chick embryos, free of infectious ALV, often contained ALV gs antigen and "type C" viruslike particles. The supposed absence of gs antibody in chickens was attributed by them to immunological tolerance caused by the endogenous gs antigen. Similar findings were later reported with murine and feline leukemia, e.g., apparently noninfectious type C particles and murine leukemia virus gs antigen are sometimes present in mice, and murine leukosis gs antibodies have not been demonstrated in mice (Geering et al., 1966). These findings, and other lines of evidence led Huebner and Todaro (1969) to formulate a general theory of carcinogenesis which postulates ubiquitous integrated RNA tumor virus genomes in vertebrates. One of the important supports for this theory was the assertion that mice, cats, and chickens are completely tolerant to the gs antigen of their homologous C-type leukemia viruses. In chickens, at least, this is not true. Perhaps the other species should be examined more carefully.

The chickens used in this study were obtained from SPAFAS, Inc. Infectious virus is seldom present in embryos from that source. Nevertheless, we previously reported a high incidence of noninfectious type C particles in these embryos (Dougherty and DiStefano, 1966; Dougherty et al., 1967). In fact, over a period of 5 years, more than 50 individual SPAFAS embryos were examined by electron microscopy, and *every one* contained viruslike C particles. The chickens used in the present study were not themselves tested (it would have required biopsy of pancreas) but we may assume from previous experience that nearly all contained particles. If this is true, then those particles did not provoke immune tolerance to ALV gs antigen. That being the case, we doubt the previous assumption, by us and others, that these particles are defective ALV. The alternate possibility, that morphologically intact avian leukosis virions contained no gs antigen, does not attract us. It was acknowledged in earlier papers (Dougherty and DiStefano, 1966; Dougherty et al., 1967) that there was no correlation between presence of gs antigen and type C particles in individual embryos and that the two might be unrelated. This now seems more likely.

In our experience approximately 50 % of embryos from SPAFAS also contain endogenous ALV gs antigen (Dougherty and DiStefano, 1966; Dougherty et al., 1967). If this is true, how do we explain the development of gs antibodies in these chickens? It may be significant that only 56 % of chickens with high titers of neutralizing, type-specific antibodies made gs CFI antibodies. Perhaps tolerance to endogenous gs antigen does develop and only those chickens that were initially free of endogenous gs antigen made gs antibodies in response to ALV infection. However, we have learned caution, and hesitate to assert on the basis of negative CFI tests that any chickens are naturally tolerant to ALV gs antigen.

There is another possibility. ALV gs antigen from virions or infected tissues is really a complex of at least 4 or 5 components (Roth and Dougherty, 1969; Armstrong, 1969; Bolognesi and Bauer, 1970; Bauer and Bolognesi, 1970). The endogenous gs antigen from uninfected chick embryos has not been obtained in sufficient quantity to determine how many or which of these components are present. Unless all gs components were present endogenously it would be possible for chickens to be tolerant to certain gs antigens and not to others. Hopefully, the immunodiffusion method could answer this question, but in practice chicken gs antibodies and endogenous gs antigen both have been too weak as immunodiffusion reagents to provide the necessary resolution of precipitin line (Roth and Dougherty, unpublished).

The possibility still exists that some chickens are naturally tolerant to some antigenic components of ALV, but this possibility remains to be proved experimentally.

ACKNOWLEDGMENT

The authors wish to acknowledge the skilled technical assistance of Miss Margaret Fatcheric.

REFERENCES

ALLEN, D. W. (1967). Zone electrophoresis of the proteins of avian myeloblastosis virus. *Biochim. Biophys. Acta* 133, 180–183.

ARMSTRONG, D. (1969). Group-specific components

of avian tumor viruses detected with chicken and hamster sera. *J. Virol.* **3**, 133–139.

BAUER, H., and BOLOGNESI, D. (1970). Polypeptides of avian RNA tumor viruses. II. Serological characterization. *Virology* **42**, 1113–1126.

BAUER, H., and JANDA, H. G. (1967). Group-specific antigen of avian leukosis-viruses. Virus specificity and relation to an antigen contained in Rous mammalian tumor cells. *Virology* **33**, 483–490.

BAUER, H., and SCHÄFER, W. (1965). Isolierung eines gruppen-spezifischen Antigens ans dem hühner-myeloblastose-virus (BAI-Stamm A). *Z. Naturforsch. B* **20**, 815–817.

BAUER, H., and SCHÄFER, W. (1966). Origin of group-specific antigen of chicken leukosis viruses. *Virology* **29**, 494–496.

BENEDICT, A. A. (1967). *In* "Methods in Immunology and Immunochemistry" (C. A. Williams and M. W. Chase, eds.), Vol. I, pp. 233–236. Academic Press, New York.

BERMAN, L. D., and SARMA, P. S. (1965). Demonstration of an avian leukosis group antigen by immunodiffusion. *Nature (London)* **207**, 263–265.

BOLOGNESI, D., and BAUER, H. (1970). Polypeptides of avian RNA tumor viruses. I. Isolation and physical and chemical analysis. *Virology* **42**, 1097–1112.

DiSTEFANO, H. S., and DOUGHERTY, R. M. (1966). Mechanisms for congenital transmission of avian leukosis virus. *J. Nat. Cancer Inst.* **37**, 869–883.

DOUGHERTY, R. M., and DiSTEFANO, H. S. (1966). Lack of relationship between infection with avian leukosis virus and presence of COFAL antigen in chick embryos. *Virology* **29**, 586–595.

DOUGHERTY, R. M., DiSTEFANO, H. S., and ROTH, F. K. (1967). Virus particles and viral antigens in chicken tissues free of infectious avian leukosis virus. *Proc. Nat. Acad. Sci. U. S.* **58**, 808–817.

DOUGHERTY, R. M., STEWART, J. A., and MORGAN, H. R. (1960). Quantitative studies of the relationships between infecting dose of Rous sarcoma virus, antiviral immune response, and tumor growth in chickens. *Virology* **11**, 349–370.

DUFF, R. G., and VOGT, P. K. (1969). Characteristics of two new avian tumor virus subgroups. *Virology* **39**, 18–30.

DULBECCO, R., VOGT, M., and STRICKLAND, A. G. (1956). A study of the basic aspects of neutralization of two animal viruses, Western equine encephalitis virus and poliomyelitis virus. *Virology* **2**, 162–205.

ECKERT, E. A., ROTT, R., and SCHÄFER, W. (1964a). Studies on the BAI strain A (avian myeloblastosis) virus. I. Production and examination of

potent virus-specific complement-fixing antiserum. *Virology* **24**, 426–433.

ECKERT, E. A., ROTT, R., and SCHÄFER, W. (1964b). Studies on the BAI strain A (avian myeloblastosis) virus. II. Some properties of the viral split products. *Virology* **24**, 434–448.

FLODIN, P., and KILLANDER, J. (1962). Fractionation of human serum proteins by gel filtration. *Biochim. Biophys. Acta* **63**, 403–410.

GEERING, G., OLD, L. J., and BOYSE, E. A. (1966). Antigens of leukemias induced by naturally occurring murine leukemia virus: their relation to antigens of Gross virus and other murine leukemia viruses. *J. Exp. Med.* **124**, 753–772.

HANAFUSA, H., and HANAFUSA, T. (1968). Further studies on RSV production from transformed cells. *Virology* **34**, 630–636.

HANAFUSA, H., HANAFUSA, T., and RUBIN, H. (1963). The defectiveness of Rous sarcoma virus. *Proc. Nat. Acad. Sci. U. S.* **49**, 572–580.

HUEBNER, R. J., ARMSTRONG, D., OKUYAN, M., SARMA, P. S., and TURNER, H. C. (1964). Specific complement-fixing viral antigens in hamster and guinea-pig tumors induced by the Schmidt-Ruppin strain of avian sarcoma. *Proc. Nat. Acad. Sci. U. S.* **51**, 742–751.

HUEBNER, R. J., ARMSTRONG, D. ROWE, W. P., TURNER, H. C., and LANE, W. T. (1963). Specific adenovirus complement-fixing viral antigens in virus-free hamster and rat tumors. *Proc. Nat. Acad. Sci. U. S.* **50**, 379–389.

HUEBNER, R. J., and TODARO, G. J. (1969). Oncogenes of RNA tumor viruses as determinants of cancer. *Proc. Nat. Acad. Sci. U. S.* **64**, 1087–1094.

ISHIZAKI, R., and VOGT, P. (1966). Immunological relationships among envelope antigens and avian tumor viruses. *Virology* **30**, 375–387.

KELLOFF, G., and VOGT, P. K. (1966). Localization of avian tumor virus group specific antigen in cell and virus. *Virology* **29**, 377–384.

MEYERS, P. (1970). Immunologic reactivity to viral antigens in chickens infected with avian leukosis viruses. Doctoral thesis. State University of New York, Upstate Medical Center, Syracuse, New York.

MEYERS, P., and DOUGHERTY, R. M. (1971). Immunologic reactivity to viral antigens in chickens infected with avian leukosis viruses. *J. Nat. Cancer Inst.* **46**, 701–711.

PAYNE, L. N., and CHUBB, R. C. (1968). Studies on the nature and genetic control of an antigen in normal chick embryos which reacts in the COFAL test. *J. Gen. Virol.* **3**, 379–391.

PAYNE, F. E., SOLOMON, J. J., and PURCHASE, H. G. (1966). Immunofluorescent studies of group-specific antigen of the avian sarcoma-leukosis viruses. *Proc. Nat. Acad. Sci. U. S.* **55**, 431–449.

RABOTTI, G. F., and BLACKHAM, E. (1970). Immunological determinants of avian sarcoma viruses: presence of group-specific antibodies in fowl sera demonstrated by complement-fixation inhibition test. *J. Nat. Cancer Inst.* **44**, 985–991.

RICE, C. E. (1948). Some factors influencing selection of complement-fixation method; parallel use of direct and indirect techniques. *J. Immunol.* **60**, 11–16.

ROTH, F. K., and DOUGHERTY, R. M. (1969). Multiple antigenic components of the group-specific antigen of avian leukosis-sarcoma viruses. *Virology* **38**, 278–284.

RUBIN, H., and VOGT, P. K. (1962). An avian leukosis virus associated with stocks of Rous sarcoma virus. *Virology* **17**, 184–194.

WEISS, R. A. (1969). Interference and neutralization studies with Bryan strain Rous sarcoma virus synthesized in the absence of helper virus. *J. Gen. Virol.* **5**, 529–539.

YOHN, D. S., WEBER, J., and McCAMMON, J. R. (1971). Avian leukosis group-specific antibodies in COFAL-negative sera. *Proc. Amer. Ass. Cancer Res.*, in press.

Immunological Determinants of Avian Sarcoma Viruses: Presence of Group-Specific Antibodies in Fowl Sera Demonstrated by Complement-Fixation Inhibition Test

G. F. RABOTTI *and* E. BLACKHAM

THE KNOWN antigenic components of the viruses of the avian leukosis complex can be summarized as follows: *a*) group-specific (gs) antigen shared by all members of the virus groups (*1, 2*) probably inside the virion (*3*); *b*) type-specific (ts) antigen at the level of the viral envelope; and *c*) transplantation antigen(s) (*4–6*) whose topographical relation to the virus (if any) is unknown.

The gs antigen is detected by its capacity to elicit complement-fixing (CF) antibodies in the sera of hamsters bearing a tumor induced by Rous sarcoma virus (RSV) (*1*). These antibodies react specifically with preparations of virus-containing (*7*) or virus-free (*8*) chick-embryo cells transformed *in vitro* by RSV or with preparations of chick fibroblasts productively infected by any of the leukosis viruses (*2*), chicken and hamster tumors induced by Schmidt-Ruppin (*1*), or Bryan high-titer strain (*9*) of RSV. These data were confirmed by immunodiffusion in agar gel (*10*). The gs antigen of the avian leukosis viruses also was demonstrated by use of sera of rabbits immunized with chemically degraded myeloblastosis virus (*3*).

These gs antibodies have not yet been demonstrated in sera of fowl bearing an RSV-induced tumor or hyperimmunized by RSV.

The ts antigen is readily shown by its capacity to induce neutralizing antibodies in the serum of the natural host of these viruses and of closely related fowl (*i.e.*, turkeys). Neutralizing antibodies are specific for each member virus of the complex and are thought to be identical to those shown by immunofluorescent tests in which chicken immune serum is used. These types of antibodies are not found in hamsters carrying an RSV-induced tumor (*11*).

The transplantation antigen(s) is demonstrated in mammals by quantitative resistance to neoplastic cell transplants in hosts previously immunized with the virus responsible for the neoplastic conversion of the transplanted cells (*4–6*). The existence of this antigen(s) in chicken tumors induced by RSV is yet to be shown.

The absence of ts antibodies in sera of hamsters carrying an RSV-induced tumor may be explained readily by the failure of the virus to synthesize the proteins of the external envelope. However, the failure to demonstrate the gs antibodies in infected chickens (the natural host) has no logical explanation. The gs antigen, specific for this group of viruses, was found in hamsters by complement-fixation and immunofluorescent tests. Chickens and related fowl do not fix guinea pig complement (*12*). Immunofluorescent tests have given negative results (*13*).

The present report describes gs antibodies in fowl sera discovered by means of a complement-fixation inhibition test. The principle of the test was to allow the interaction between an avian sarcoma antigen (from infected chicken fibroblast cultures, chicken tumors, or hamster tumors) and the immune fowl serum. This interaction would then prevent the fixation of added complement in the presence of hamster serum

169

immune to the Schmidt-Ruppin strain of RSV, because the antigen would no longer be available for the reaction.

MATERIALS AND METHODS

Strains of viruses.—The following strains were used to infect *in vitro* fowl fibroblasts and to induce tumors in fowl and hamsters: *a*) Byran high-titer strain, type A [BH-RSV (RAV-1)] (*14*); *b*) Schmidt-Ruppin strain which was found not to form foci on K/2 type of chicken fibroblasts and was designated accordingly (*14*) SR-RSV, type B; *c*) Harris strain (H-RSV), type A; and *d*) the strain of avian lymphomatosis RPL12 (wild strain).

Cell cultures.—Chicken-embryo fibroblast cultures were prepared by standard methods and infected in large bottles with the different strains of RSV at a moiety of 10. Uninfected cultures were used as controls. The fecundated hen's eggs free of the resistance-inducing factor (RIF) were obtained from Dr. R. E. Luginbuhl, University of Connecticut, Storrs, Connecticut.

Japanese quail fibroblast cultures were prepared similarly and infected with different strains of RSV, also at a moiety of 10. Uninfected cultures were used as controls. The embryonated quail eggs were obtained from the Germfree Life Research Center, Tampa, Florida.

Virus assay.—The RSV inocula were titrated by the standard *in vitro* method (*15*) with the use of chicken fibroblast cultures. The lymphomatosis virus was assayed by the COFAL method (*2*), the gs complement-fixation test for avian leukosis.

Neutralization test.—Tenfold dilutions of the control and immune fowl antisera were made with the use of tissue culture medium. The antisera were incubated with 100 focus-forming units (FFU) of the different strains of RSV for 40 minutes at 37°C; 0.1 ml of each mixture was then used to infect 2 dishes of secondary chick-embryo fibroblast cultures. The titer was the reciprocal of the highest dilution of antiserum inhibiting 90% of the foci.

Tumors.—Sarcomas were induced in fowl by wing-web inoculation of 0.2 ml of cell-free preparations containing 10^6 FFU of the virus. Tumors were harvested from chickens 9 days post inoculation and from turkeys and Japanese quail 14 days post inoculation. They were induced in newborn hamsters by subcutaneous inoculation of 0.1 ml cell-free preparations containing 10^7 FFU of BH-RSV or 10^6 SR-RSV. All tumors were preserved at $-70°C$.

Preparation of antigens.—The antigen was prepared from tissue cultures infected 16–20 days previously. At that time, the corresponding uninfected cultures were also harvested. The infected and control cells were packed by centrifugation and resuspended in 10% (v/v) of the original tissue culture medium. The preparations were then frozen at $-60°C$ and thawed. This procedure was done 3 times, and the suspension was kept frozen at $-60°C$.

Tumors were processed similarly by homogenization in 20% (v/v) of tumors in Eagle's basal medium.

Before use, tissue culture and tumor antigen preparations were spun at $2000 \times g$ for 20 minutes in a refrigerated centrifuge.

Preparation of antisera.—Antisera were prepared in chickens and turkeys about 2 months old. Fowl surviving wing-web inoculation of 10^3 FFU of RSV were hyperimmunized with 5×10^5 FFU of the same strain of virus weekly for 4 weeks. They were bled by heart puncture 2 weeks after the last inoculation.

Sera were collected from hamsters bearing large primary tumors induced by SR-RSV.

The potency of the individual chicken and turkey sera was assayed by the neutralization test. Only antisera showing titers of 1:256 or more in chickens and 1:128 or more in turkeys were used. Some sera also were tested in standard tissue culture (*16*) for neutralizing antibodies to influenza A, B, and C, mumps, Newcastle disease virus, and pox influenza 1, 2, 3, and 4; they were found to be negative. A total of 27 immune and 4 control

171

chicken sera and 16 immune and 2 control turkey sera were tested by complement-fixation inhibition. Individual sera from hamsters bearing a primary SR-RSV-induced tumor were checked by the complement-fixation test, as described by Huebner *et al.* (*1*) with the microtechnique of Sever (*17*).

Several positive hamster sera were pooled. This serum pool had a titer of 1:320 against 4 U of SR-RSV antigen from a wing-web tumor. It was negative for CF antibodies against adenovirus types 7 and 12, simian virus 40, polyoma hamster tumor antigens, and control, uninoculated tissue-culture preparations of RIF-free, chick-embryo fibroblasts. It was also negative for neutralizing antibodies to BH-RSV or SR-RSV.

Complement-fixation inhibition tests.—All tests were done in plastic plates, with the microtechnique of Sever (*17*) used.

Before each test, chicken, turkey, and hamster sera were heat inactivated at 56°C for 30 minutes.

For preliminary standardizations of all antigens used, the highest dilution of antigen was determined that still gave a 4+ reaction in the standard (*1*) complement-fixation test using 4 U of complement and 1:80 dilution of the RSV-immune hamster serum pool set as a standard in this laboratory. A few antigens had moderate anticomplementary activity in both normal and infected chicken cells. These antigens were not used in the complement-fixation inhibition test.

All the decomplemented immune sera of fowl were tested by complement fixation against all RSV antigen preparations, in chessboard-type reactions, and were found to be negative.

For the complement-fixation inhibition test, 4 U of antigen was then incubated with twofold dilutions of fowl antisera at 37°C for 2 hours. All the wells then received the hamster immune serum (dilution 1:80) and 2 U of guinea pig complement. After the plates were incubated overnight at 4°C, the indicator system was added.

All tests included the following controls: known positive and negative antigens, known negative hamster serum, negative chicken serum, test for anticomplementary activity, 4 tubes for complement control (back-titration), and test for sheep cell fragility.

The titer of the complement-fixation inhibition test was expressed as the reciprocal of the highest dilution of fowl antiserum capable of binding the antigen and inhibiting the fixation of the complement by the hamster serum. This was expressed by the wells containing the highest dilution of fowl sera in which complete hemolysis occurred.

RESULTS

Demonstration, by Complement-Fixation Inhibition Test, of Specific Antibodies in Sera of RSV-Immune Fowl Against RSV Antigens From Tissue Cultures

Table 1 shows representative reactions, in the complement-fixation inhibition test, of chicken immune sera against antigens from chicken fibroblasts infected *in vitro* by the virus homologous to the antiserum. The antibody titer was 8–32 for most sera. The normal tissue culture antigens did not react. Comparable results are shown in table 2, where the antigen preparations were chicken and hamster sarcomas. Immune sera from turkeys reacted in the same manner (table 3). The titer of gs antibodies showed no differences in sera of immunized fowl with or without a tumor.

Group Reactivity of RSV-Immune Fowl Sera

As measured by the complement-fixation inhibition test, broad cross reactivity was evident in RSV-immune sera of chickens and turkeys against all the RSV antigen tested (table 4).

Table 5 shows the results when the antigen was prepared in turkeys and in Japanese quail. The results were similar to those obtained with antigens prepared in chickens.

Antisera prepared in Japanese quail were not available.

173

TABLE 1.—Chessboard reactions, in complement-fixation inhibition test, between representative sera of RSV-immune chicken and RSV antigens prepared in tissue cultures*

Chicken serum dilution†

Band 1 — Antigen: CEF,‡ Infected, BH-RSV (RAV 1)

Antigen dilution†	BH-RSV (A)					BH-RSV (B)					BH-RSV (C)				
	4	8	16	32	64	4	8	16	32	64	4	8	16	32	64
4	4§	2	4	0	0	4	0	3	0	0	4	0	0	0	0
8	4	4	4	3	0	0	0	0	0	0	2	2	2	2	2
16	4	4	4	4	2	3	0	0	0	0	4	2	2	2	2
32	4	4	4	4	4	4	4	4	4	4	4	4	4	4	4

Band 2 — Antigen: CEF,‡ Infected, SR-RSV (type B)

Antigen dilution†	SR-RSV (A)					SR-RSV (B)					SR-RSV (C)				
	4	8	16	32	64	4	8	16	32	64	4	8	16	32	64
4	2	0	0	0	0	0	0	0	0	0	2	0	0	0	0
8	4	4	2	2	0	2	2	2	2	2	4	2	2	2	2
16	4	4	4	4	4	4	4	4	4	2	4	4	4	4	4
32	4	4	4	4	4	4	4	4	4	4	4	4	4	4	4

Band 3 — Antigen: CEF,‡ Infected, H-RSV (type A)

Antigen dilution†	H-RSV (A)					H-RSV (B)									
	4	8	16	32	64	4	8	16	32	64					
4	4	2	0	0	0	0	0	0	0	0	Not tested				
8	4	4	4	2	0	2	2	2	2	2					
16	4	4	4	4	4	4	4	4	2	0					
32	4	4	4	4	4	4	4	4	4	4					

*With normal chicken serum (no neutralizing antibodies at 1:4 dilution), no hemolysis was observed. All the reactions were carried out with addition of 1:80 dilution of SR-RSV-immune hamster serum (see text).

†Reciprocal of dilution.

‡RIF-free chick-embryo fibroblast cultures.

§Hemolysis, reading scale of 0–4.

TABLE 2.—Reactions, in complement-fixation inhibition test, of avian and hamster sarcoma antigens with representative pools of immune chicken sera

Antigens	Chicken serum titers*	
	Immune	Control
BH-RSV		
Chicken tumor	16†–64	≤ 4
Hamster tumor	8–32	≤ 4
Tissue-culture hamster-tumor cells	8–32	< 4
SR-RSV		
Chicken tumor	8–64	≤ 4
Hamster tumor	8–32	≤ 4
Tissue-culture hamster-tumor cells	8–32	< 4
H-RSV		
Chicken tumor	8–32	≤ 4
Hamster tumor	4–16	≤ 4
Tissue-culture hamster-tumor cells	4–16	< 4

*Total number of sera examined: BH-RSV = 3, SR-RSV = 7, and H-RSV = 2.
†Reciprocal of dilution.

TABLE 3.—Reaction, in complement-fixation inhibition test, of avian and hamster sarcoma antigens with representative pools of turkey sera immunized with BH-RSV

Antigens	Turkey serum titers*	
	Immune	Normal control
Chicken tumor (BH-RSV)	16†–64	≤ 4
CEF‡ tissue culture (BH-RSV)	8–16	≤ 4
Hamster tumor (SR-RSV)	4–16	≤ 4
Tissue-culture hamster-tumor cells (SR-RSV)	4–8	< 4

*Total number of sera examined: 16.
†Reciprocal of dilution.
‡RIF-free chick-embryo fibroblast cultures.

TABLE 4.—Group reactivity, in complement-fixation inhibition test, between RSV-immune fowl sera and avian leukosis antigens prepared in chickens and hamsters

Antigens	Fowl serum titers*			
	Chicken			Turkey
	BH-RSV	SR-RSV	H-RSV	BH-RSV
BH-RSV				
Chicken tumor	16†-64	8-64	8-32	16-64
Tissue culture CEF‡	32-64	16-64	16-64	32-64
Hamster tumor	8-32	8-32	4-16	4-16
Tissue-culture hamster-tumor cells	8-32	8-32	4-16	4-16
SR-RSV				
Chicken tumor	8-64	8-64	8-16	8-32
Tissue culture CEF	16-64	4-32	16-32	4-16
Hamster tumor	8-32	4-16	4-16	8-16
Tissue-culture hamster-tumor cells	8-32	4-16	4-16	4-8
H-RSV				
Chicken tumor	8-16	4-32	8-16	4-16
Tissue culture CEF	4-32	8-16	4-16	4-8
Hamster tumor	8-16	4-16	4-8	8-16
Tissue-culture hamster-tumor cells	8-16	8-16	8-16	8-32
RPL12				
Tissue culture CEF	4-16	8-16	4-32	8-32

*Total number of sera examined: 34.
†Reciprocal of dilution.
‡RIF-free chick-embryo fibroblast cultures.

Comparison of Titers of gs Antibodies Versus ts Antibodies in Representative Sera

The titer of gs antibodies in chicken and turkey sera was significantly lower than that of ts antibodies in the same serum. Table 6 shows the values of the 2 types of antibodies measured in a representative number of chicken and turkey sera. All fowl sera with neutralizing antibodies of 1:256 or more showed gs antibodies. Nevertheless, no correlation between the 2 types of antibody in the same serum specimen was found.

Comparison of Titers of gs Antibodies in Fowl and Tumor-Bearing Hamsters

In chicken and turkey sera with high titers of neutralizing antibodies (1:512 or more), the titer of gs antibodies never exceeded 1:64. But the titer of gs antibodies in hamsters with SR-RSV-induced tumors reached occasionally 1:512.

DISCUSSION

The presence of gs antibodies in fowl immunized with different strains of RSV has been shown. The type specificity of the various antisera demonstrated by the neutralization test agrees with previous

TABLE 5.—Cross reactivity, in complement-fixation inhibition test, between RSV antigens produced in turkeys and Japanese quail and RSV-immune chicken sera.

Antigen	Chicken serum titers	
	BH-RSV	SR-RSV
BH-RSV		
Turkey tumor	16–64	8–32
Japanese quail tumor	8–32	4–16
SR-RSV		
Turkey tumor	4–16	8–32
Japanese quail tumor	8–16	4–16

TABLE 6.—Comparison of titers of gs and ts (neutralizing) antibodies in representative individual fowl sera

Sera		gs antibody titers against antigens from tissue culture			Titers of neutralizing antibodies versus 100 FFU of virus		
		BH-RSV	SR-RSV	H-RSV	BR-RSV	SR-RSV	H-RSV
Antigens:							
Chicken							
BH-RSV	(8)	32	32	8	256	<4	<4
BH-RSV	(7)	64	16	8	256	<4	<4
BH-RSV	(14)	32	16	4	512	<4	<4
SR-RSV	(1)	32	16	4	<4	512	<4
SR-RSV	(9)	16	16	8	<4	512	<4
H-RSV	(5)	16	16	8	<4	<4	256
Antigens:							
Turkeys							
BH-RSV	(72)	64	64	32	128	<4	—
BH-RSV	(78)	64	32	16	256	<4	—
SR-RSV	(81)	32	32	16	<4	256	—

findings (*18, 19*) and excludes the possibility of cross contamination between the different strains used in these experiments. The absence of cross reaction in neutralization tests also shows that the gs antibodies in fowl sera have no neutralizing activity. CF sera from hamsters carrying an SR-RSV-induced tumor also show no neutralizing activity (*11*). The biological similarity between gs antibodies in fowl and hamster sera is therefore evident.

A difference between gs antibodies in fowl and hamsters is in their titers in the sera. Titers are frequently high in hamsters but are never high in fowl. Being of quantitative order, this difference needs, however, to be regarded with some caution, since the gs antibodies are measured in the two animal species by operationally different methods.

Data obtained by the immunofluorescent technique (*13*) suggest that chicken immune sera prepared against avian tumor viruses lack gs-reactive antibodies. From our findings, the failure to demonstrate, with immunocytological methods, the RSV gs antibodies in fowl sera may be related to low titer. If so, selecting the proper concentration of chicken antisera could demonstrate by immunofluorescence the gs antigen in chickens productively infected with avian tumor viruses and in so-called nonproducer cells.

The presence of an RSV-specific antigen in RSV-induced meningeal tumor cells of dogs has been demonstrated by immunofluorescence (*20*). In those tests, chicken immune serum anti-BH-RSV was used. The presence of the antigen in dog tumors induced with different strains of RSV suggested a group reactivity.

The results of the present investigations confirm and clarify those early findings.

REFERENCES

(*1*) HUEBNER RJ, ROWE WP, TURNER HC, et al: Specific adenovirus complement-fixing antigens in virus-free hamster and rat tumors. Proc Nat Acad Sci USA 50:379–389, 1963

(2) SARMA PS, TURNER HC, HUEBNER RJ: An avian leucosis group-specific complement fixation reaction. Application for the detection and assay of non-cytopathogenic leucosis viruses. Virology 23: 313–321, 1964

(3) BAUER H, SCHÄFER W: Origin of group-specific antigen of chicken leukosis viruses. Virology 29:494–497, 1966

(4) SJÖGREN HO, JONSSON N: Resistance against iso-transplantation of mouse tumors induced by Rous sarcoma virus. Exp Cell Res 32:618–621, 1963

(5) HARRIS, RJC, CHESTERMAN FC: Growth of Rous sarcoma in rats, ferrets, and hamsters. Nat Cancer Inst Monogr 17:321–335, 1964

(6) SVOBODA J: Antitumor immunity against RSV-induced tumors in mammals. In Specific Tumor Antigens (Harris RJC, ed.), vol 2. Un Int Contra Cancr Monograph Series. Munskgaard, Copenhagen, 1967, pp 133–146

(7) ARMSTRONG D, OKUYAN M, HUEBNER RJ: Complement-fixing antigens in tissue cultures of avian leucosis viruses. Science 144:1584, 1964

(8) VOGT PK, SARMA PS, HUEBNER RJ: Presence of avian tumor virus group-specific antigen in nonproducing Rous sarcoma cells of the chicken. Virology 27:233–236, 1965

(9) CASEY, MJ, RABOTTI GF, SARMA PS, et al: Complement-fixing antigens in hamster tumors induced by the Bryan strain of Rous sarcoma virus. Science 151: 1086–1088, 1966

(10) BERMAN LD, SARMA PS: Demonstration of an avian leucosis group antigen by immunodiffusion. Nature (London) 207:263–265, 1965

(11) HUEBNER RJ, ARMSTRONG D, OKUYAN M, et al: Specific complement-fixing viral antigens in hamster and guinea pig tumors induced by the Schmidt-Ruppin strain of avian sarcoma. Proc Nat Acad Sci USA 51:742–750, 1964

(12) FULTON F: The measurement of complement-fixation by viruses. Advances Virus Res 5: 247–287, 1958

(13) KELLOFF G, VOGT P: Localization of avian tumor virus group-specific antigen in cell and virus. Virology 29:377–384, 1966

(14) VOGT PK, ISHIZAKI R: Patterns of viral interference in the avian leukosis and sarcoma complex. Virology 30:368–374, 1966

(15) TEMIN HM, RUBIN H: Characteristics of an assay for Rous sarcoma virus and Rous sarcoma cells in tissue culture. Virology 5:669–688, 1958

(16) COOK MK, ANDREWS BE, FOX, HH, et al: Antigenic relationship among the "newer" myxoviruses (para influenza). Amer J Hyg 69:250–264, 1959

(*17*) SEVER JL: Application of a microtechnique to viral serological investigation. J Immun 88:320–329, 1962

(*18*) SIMONS PJ, DOUGHERTY RM: Antigenic characteristics of three variants of Rous sarcoma virus. J Nat Cancer Inst 31:1275–1283, 1963

(*19*) SARMA PS, HUEBNER RJ, ARMSTRONG D: A simplified tissue culture tube neutralization test for Rous sarcoma virus antibodies. Proc Soc Exp Biol Med 115: 481–486, 1964

(*20*) RABOTTI GF, BUCCIARELLI E, DALTON AJ: Presence of particles with the morphology of viruses of the avian leukosis complex in meningeal tumors induced in dogs by Rous sarcoma virus. Virology 29:684–686, 1966

Cutaneous skin test for delayed hypersensitivity in hamsters to viral induced tumor antigens[1]

RICHARD G. OLSEN, JAMES R. McCAMMON, JOSEPH WEBER, AND DAVID S. YOHN

The cell-mediated immune response is now recognized by many investigators (1) as playing a determining role in the hosts immunologic defense against oncogenesis. In vitro means to monitor cell-mediated immunity have included macrophage inhibition (3), cytotoxicity (7), and colony inhibition (4). These procedures have not always correlated with in vivo observations. Consequently many studies continue to rely on specific delayed-type hypersensitivity reactions in vivo (2, 5).

Since the hamster is commonly used as a model system in experimental viral oncology it was of interest to determine whether a similar specific skin test response could be monitored in this laboratory animal to DNA and RNA virus induced tumor antigens.

The hamster tumors used in this study were induced with adenovirus type-12 (Ad-12), Rous Sarcoma Virus, Schmidt-Rupin strain (RSV-SR), and SV40 virus or SV40 DNA. The Ad-12 tumors were from a transplantable line described previously (9). The RSV-SR tumors were transplanted at 3- to 4-week intervals in weanling PD-4 inbred hamsters, while primary SV40 tumors were induced in random bred hamsters. For preparation of skin test antigens, RSV-SR

tumors were homogenized in an equal volume of Hanks' balanced salt solution (H-BSS), clarified by centrifugation, and subsequently precipitated with 2 M neutral ammonium sulphate. The precipitate was dissolved in distilled water and dialyzed against distilled water. The final preparation contained about 16 units of COFAL antigen per milliliter and about 4.6 mg protein/ml.

Ad-12 transplantable tumors and SV-40 primary tumors were freed of necrotic material, washed, minced finely, and placed in equal volume of H-BSS. This material was subsequently sonicated in an ice bath at 20 kc/s for 4 min. The Ad-12 preparation contained about 64 units of complement-fixing T-antigen per milliliter and about 42 mg protein/ml.

Skin test procedure consisted of removing the hair by shaving followed by skin testing intradermally with 0.05 ml of appropriate antigens. Skin tests were considered positive if they developed 16–48 h postinoculation and if the erythema and induration were larger than 4.0 mm. The gross appearance and histopathology of the positive skin tests in hamsters were similar to that described by Ramseier and Billingham (6).

In the RSV-SR, Ad-12, and SV-40 tumor systems the immunologic specificity of the skin test was determined by testing tumor-bearing hamsters with homologous and heterologous tumor antigens simultaneously.

[1]This study was supported in part by National Institutes of Health Contract No. 69-2233 from the Special Virus Cancer Program of the National Cancer Institute.

182

Of 39 Ad-12 tumor bearing inbred hamsters, 36 reacted to Ad-12 tumor antigen and none to SV-40 tumor antigens (Table 1). One of 16 Ad-12 tumor bearing hamsters tested reacted with RSV-SR tumor antigen whereas balanced salt solution failed to elicit a positive skin test in these animals.

Of 77 inbred hamsters bearing RSV-SR tumors 60 gave a positive delayed-type skin test to RSV-SR tumor antigens. In this group only 1 out of 77 cross-reacted with Ad-12 antigen and none reacted with balanced salt solution control antigen.

Skin tests on non-tumor bearing hamsters revealed no reaction with Ad-12 tumor antigens in 25 animals tested; no reaction in 10 animals tested with SV-40 antigens and no reaction in 17 animals tested with balanced salt solution. RSV-SR antigens gave a false positive response in one of the seven non-tumor bearing animals.

The skin test was used to determine the onset of delayed-type immune response following tumor challenge. Ad-12 and RSV-SR tumor bearing hamsters developed positive delayed-type skin test to homologous antigen at the time tumors became palpable (Table 2). The earliest positive skin test appeared two weeks after inoculation with tumor. All but one positive animal converted by the fifth or sixth week. With one exception the non-tumor-bearing control hamsters that were skin-tested each week remained negative during the 6-week experimental period, demonstrating that the skin test antigen did not readily sensitize the animals.

No generalization can be made about the extent of the skin test response and the size of tumor in either the RSV or Ad-12 experiments. It should be emphasized, however, that the skin test response did not diminish as the tumor increased in mass. Rats with tumors, induced by benzypyrene (8), developed a positive skin test only if macroscopic amounts of tumor were removed; thus it was proposed that the immune response was exhausted by large tumor masses.

The use of inbred hamsters in our experiments precluded the possibility of histocompatibility reactions. The absence of a positive skin test by Ad-12 and RSV-SR tumor bearing hamsters to SV40 tumor antigen, which was prepared from tumors induced in random bred hamsters,

TABLE 1

Delayed-type hypersensitivity reactions induced in the skin of hamsters bearing virus-induced transplanted tumors

Source of skin test antigen	Delayed-type hypersensitivity skin reactions in hamsters with:			
	Ad-12 tumor	RSV-SR tumor	SV-40 tumor	No tumor
Ad-12 hamster tumor (PD-4)	36/39[a]	1/77	0/8	0/25
RSV-SR hamster tumor (PD-4)	1/16	60/77	n.t.	1/7
SV-40 hamster tumor (random-bred)	0/39	n.t.	4/8	0/10
Control-balanced salt solution	0/16	0/77	0/8	0/17

[a]Number positive over number tested.
Note: n.t. = not tested.

TABLE 2

Time course of development of delayed-type hypersensitivity in hamsters to tumor antigens found in Ad-12 and Rous virus induced transplantable tumors

Weeks after tumor transplantation	Positive delayed-type skin reactions/number of hamsters with tumors/number of hamsters transplanted with		No tumor (controls) but skin tested with:	
	Ad-12 tumor	RSV-SR tumor	Ad-12 Ag	RSV-SR Ag
0	0/0/5	0/0/9	0/0/5	0/0/4
1	0/0/5	0/0/9	0/0/5	0/0/4
2	2/1/5	n.t.	0/0/5	n.t.
3	3/3/5	4/5/9	0/0/5	0/0/4
4	4/4/5	n.t.	0/0/5	n.t.
5	5/5/5	n.t.	0/0/5	n.t.
6	5/5/5	6/7/7	1/0/5	0/0/4

183

further indicates that histocompatibility antigens were not responsible for these reactions.

The nature of the antigens in the RSV and Ad-12 systems which elicited the positive skin test response is uncertain. The Ad-12 tumor contained T-antigen and tumor specific transplantation antigen (TSTA). The RSV tumor contained avian leukosis group specific antigens; TSTA antigens were probably present. Experiments are being conducted to ascertain whether the skin test can be used to detect a response to Ad-12 TSTA antigens.

1. ALLISON, H. D. 1967. Cell mediated immune responses to virus infections and virus induced tumors. Brit. Med. Bull. 23: 60–65.
2. CHURCHILL, W. H., JR., H. U. RAPP, B. S. KRONMAN, and T. BORSOS. 1968. Detection of antigens of a new diethylnitrosomine-induced transplantable hepatoma by delayed hypersensitivity. J. Nat. Cancer Inst. 41: 13–29.
3. GEORGE, M., and J. H. VAUGHN. 1962. In vitro cell migration as a model for delayed hypersensitivity. Proc. Soc. Exp. Biol. Med. 11: 514.
4. HELLSTRÖM, I. 1967. A colony inhibition (CT) technique for demonstration of tumor cell destruction by lymphoid cells in vitro. Int. J. Cancer, 2: 65–68.
5. HOLLINSHEAD, A., D. GLEN, B. BUNNAG, P. GOLD, and R. HERBERMAN. 1970. Skin-reactive soluble antigen from intestinal cancer-cell membranes and relationship to carcinoembryonic antigens. Lancet, 6: 1191–1195.
6. RAMSEIER, J., and R. E. BILLINGHAM. 1964. Delayed cutaneous hypersensitivity reactions and transplantation immunity in syrian hamster. Ann. N.Y. Acad. Sci. 120: 379–392.
7. RUDDLE, N. H., and B. H. WAKSMAN. 1967. Cytotoxic effect of lymphocyte-antigen interaction in delayed hypersensitivity. Science (Washington), 157: 1060.
8. WANG, M. 1968. Delayed hypersensitivity to extracts from primary sarcomata in the autochthonous host. Int. J. Cancer, 3: 483–490.
9. YOHN, D. S., L. WEISS, and M. E. NEIDERS. 1968. A comparison of the distribution of tumors produced by intravenous injection of type 12 Adenovirus and Adeno-12 tumor cells. Cancer Res. 28: 571–576.

AUTHOR INDEX

KEY-WORD TITLE INDEX

DATE DUE

DEMCO 38-297